A Picture Book Of Raindrops & Rainbows

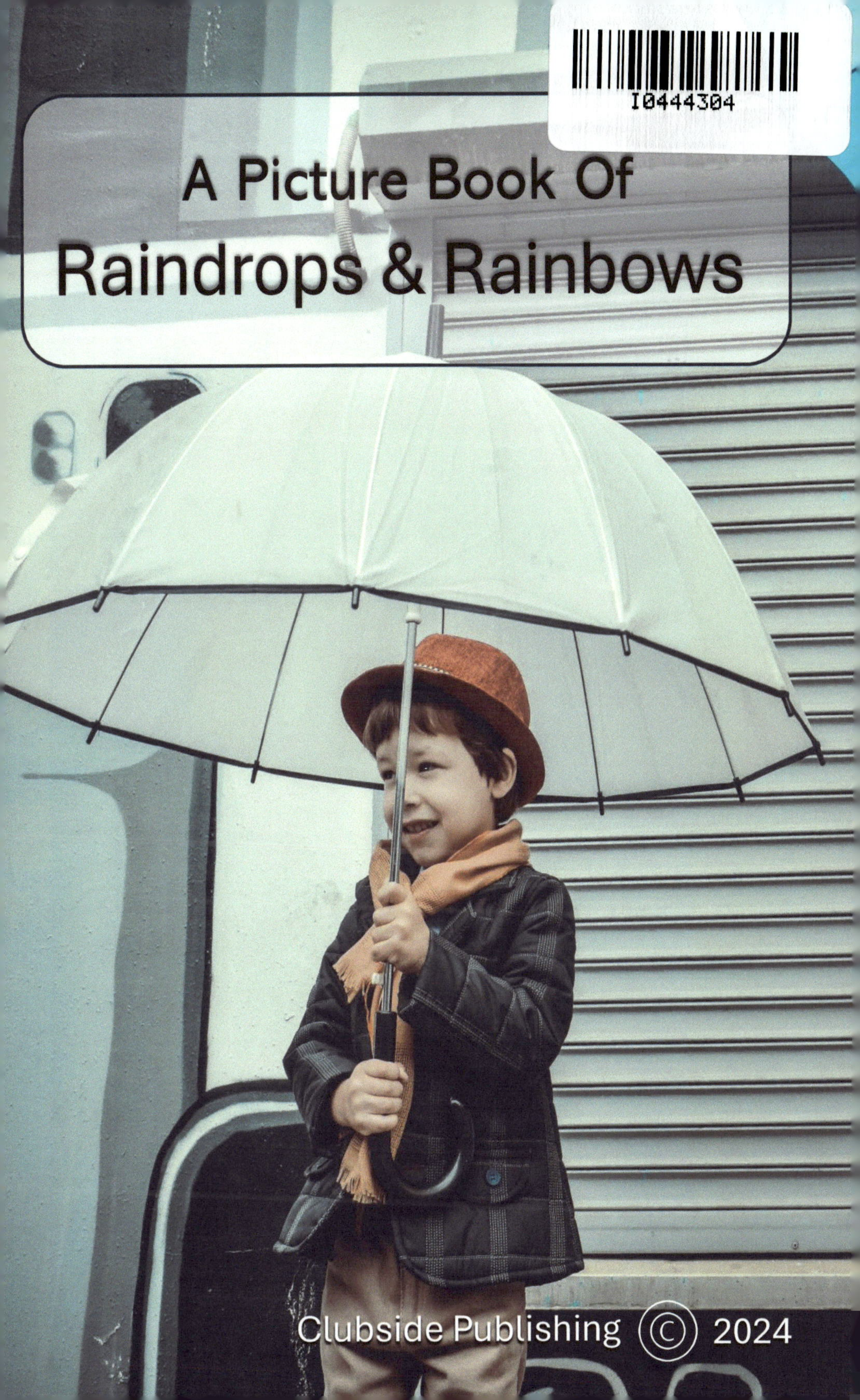

Clubside Publishing © 2024

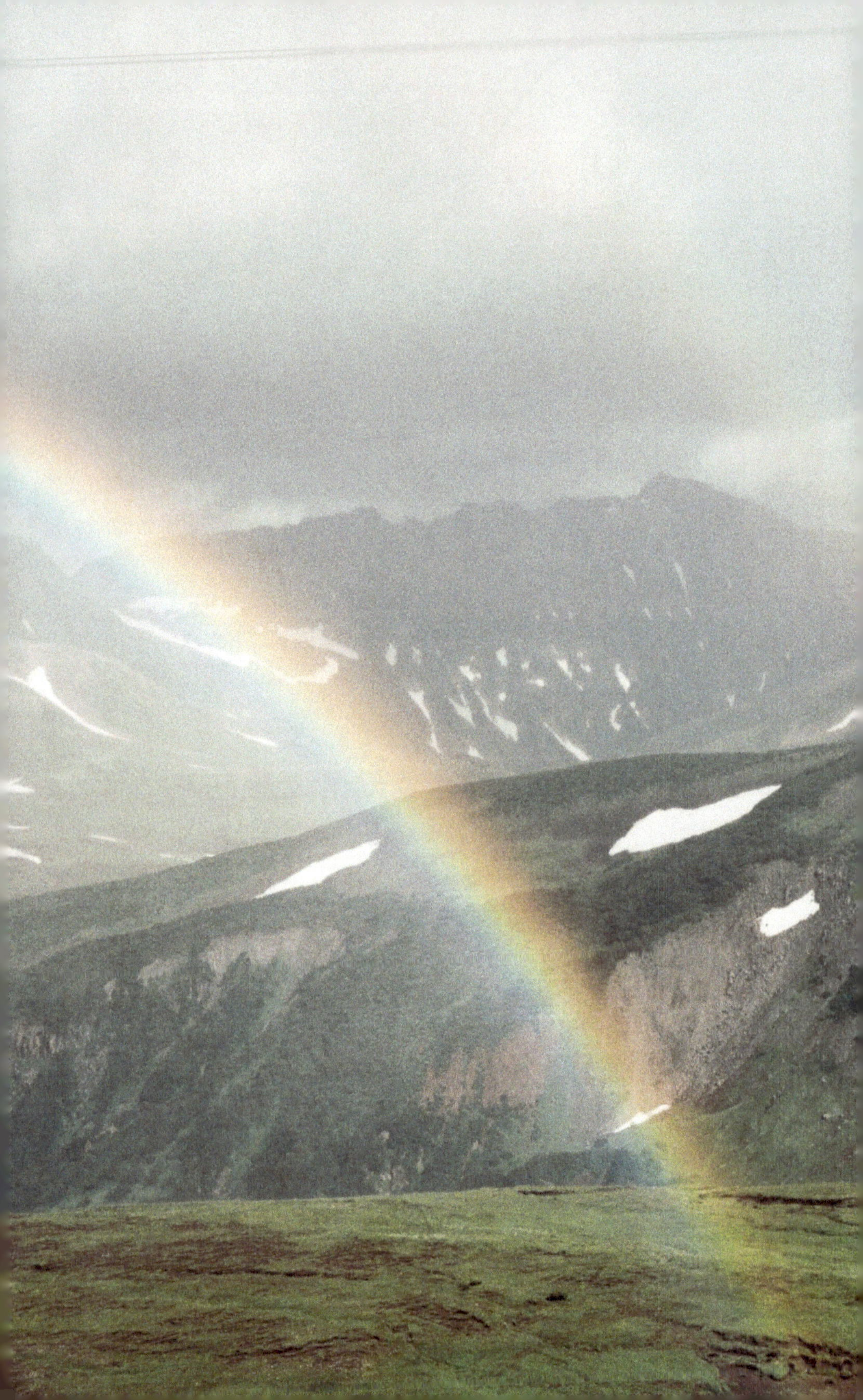

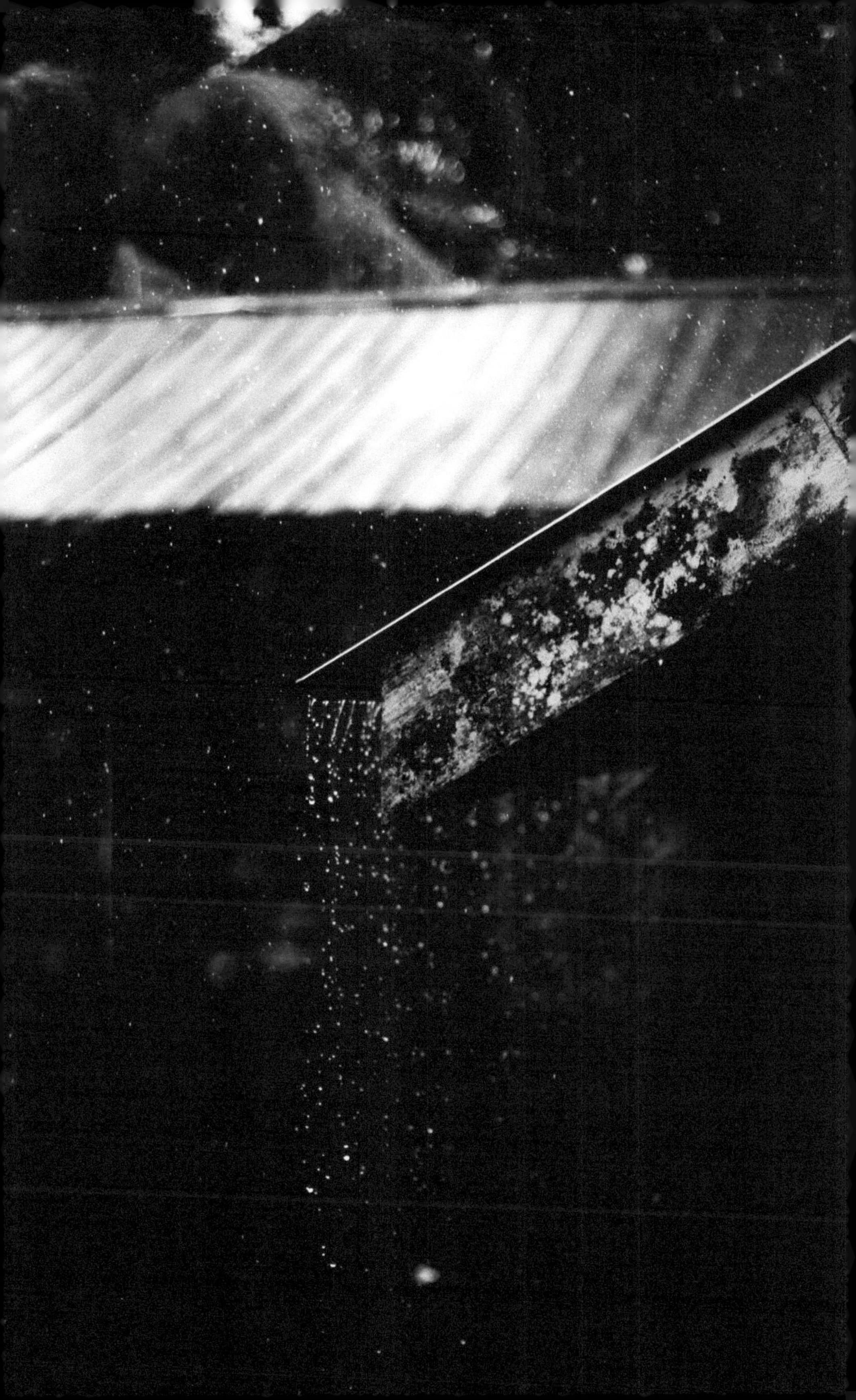

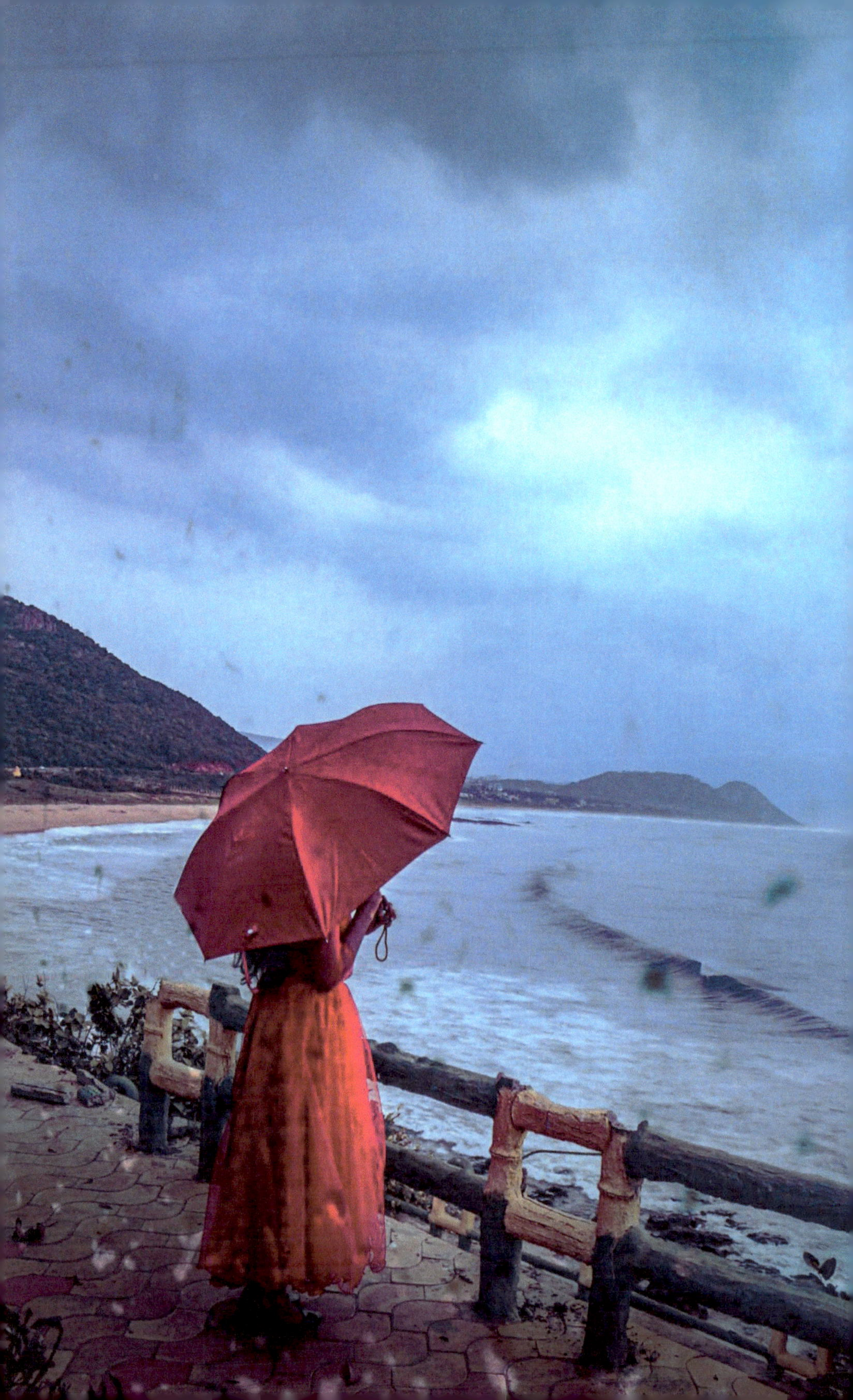

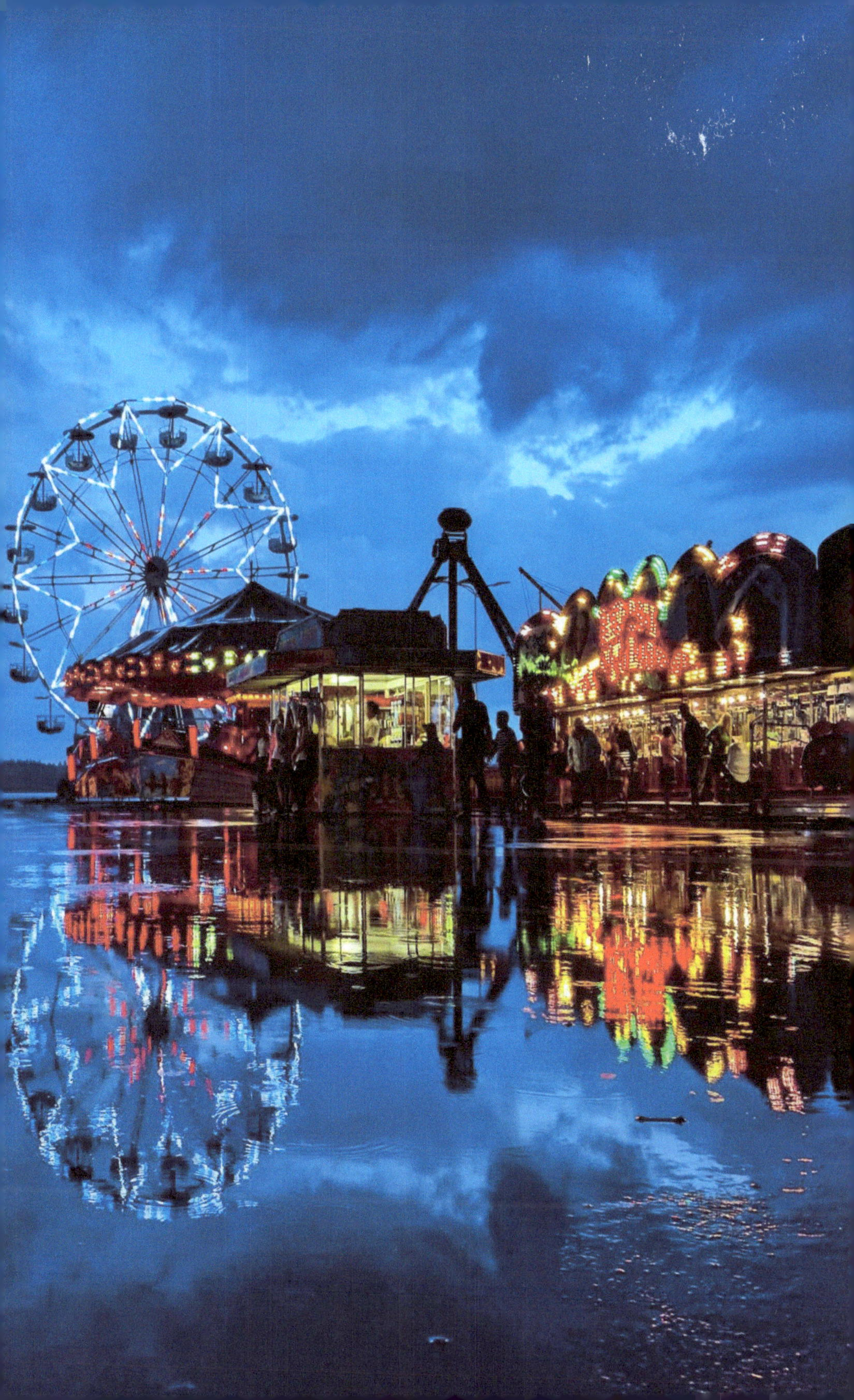

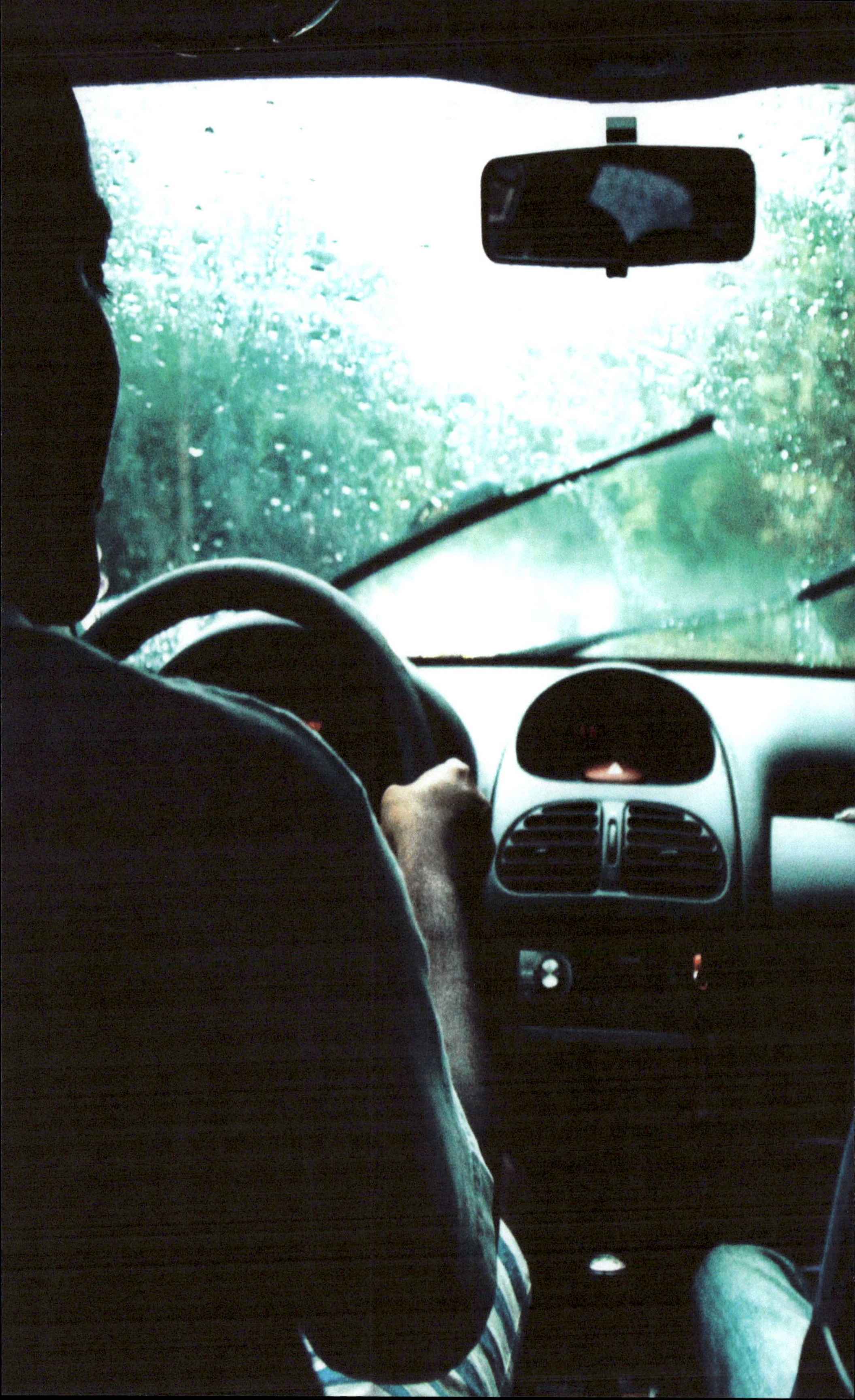

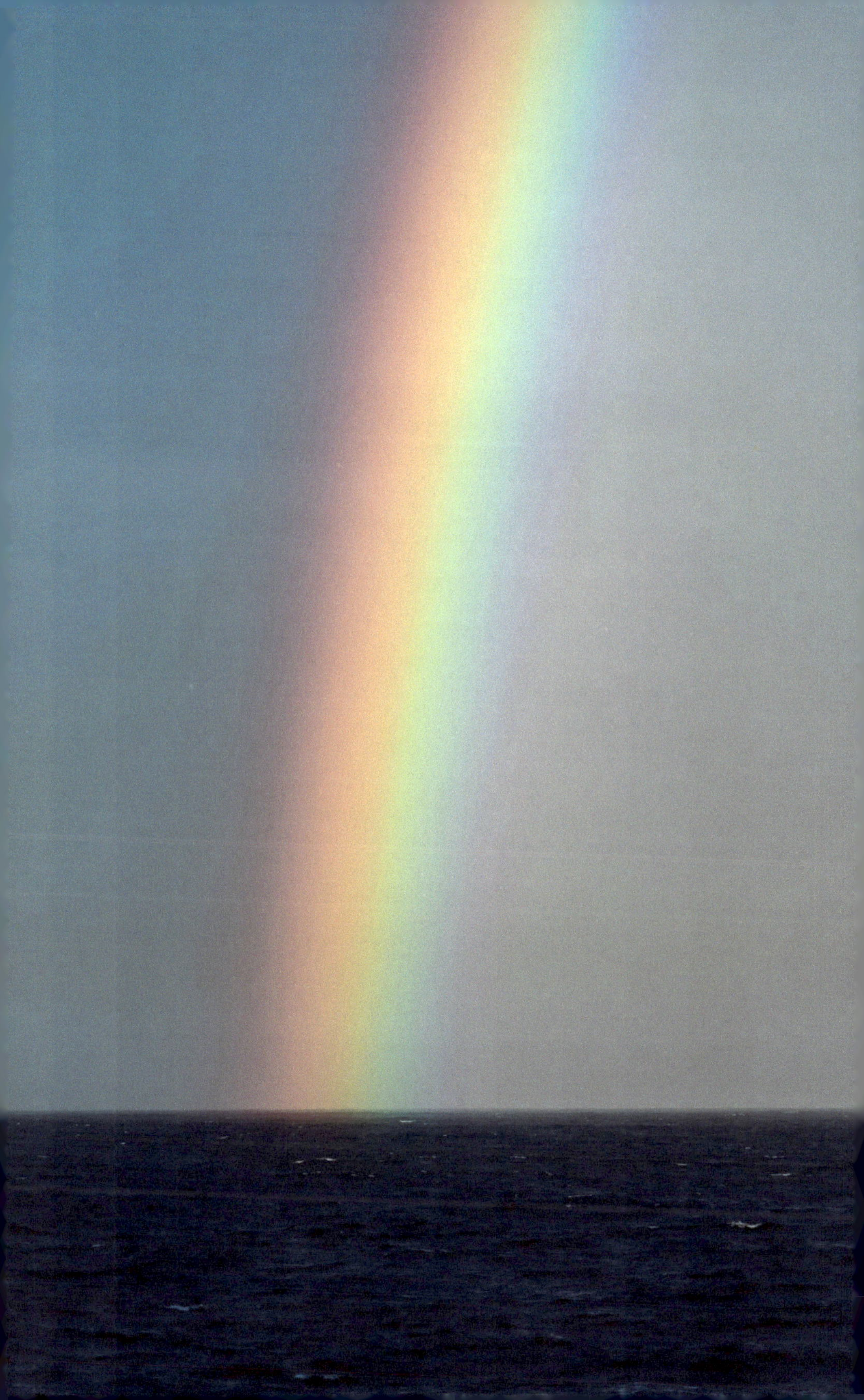

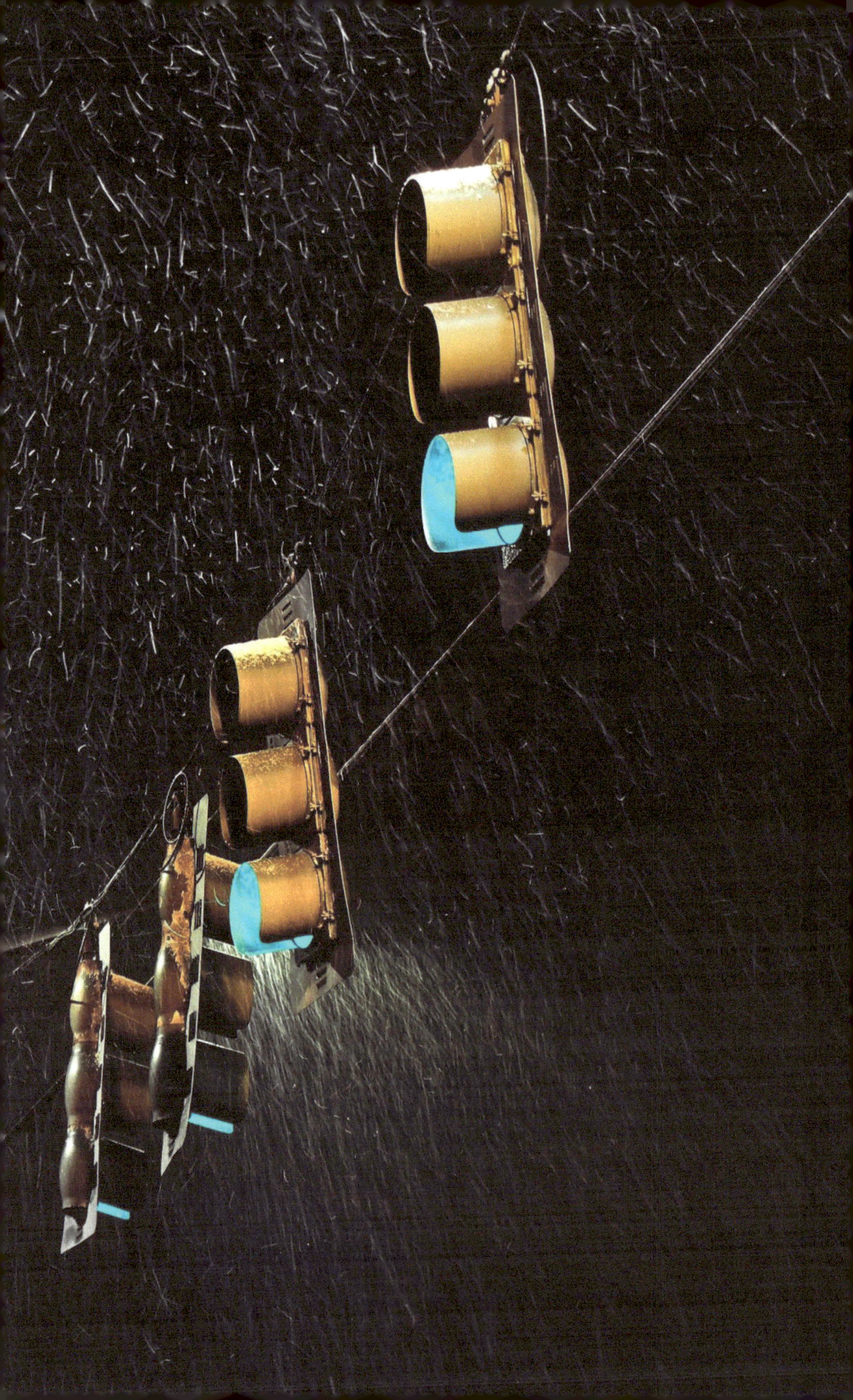

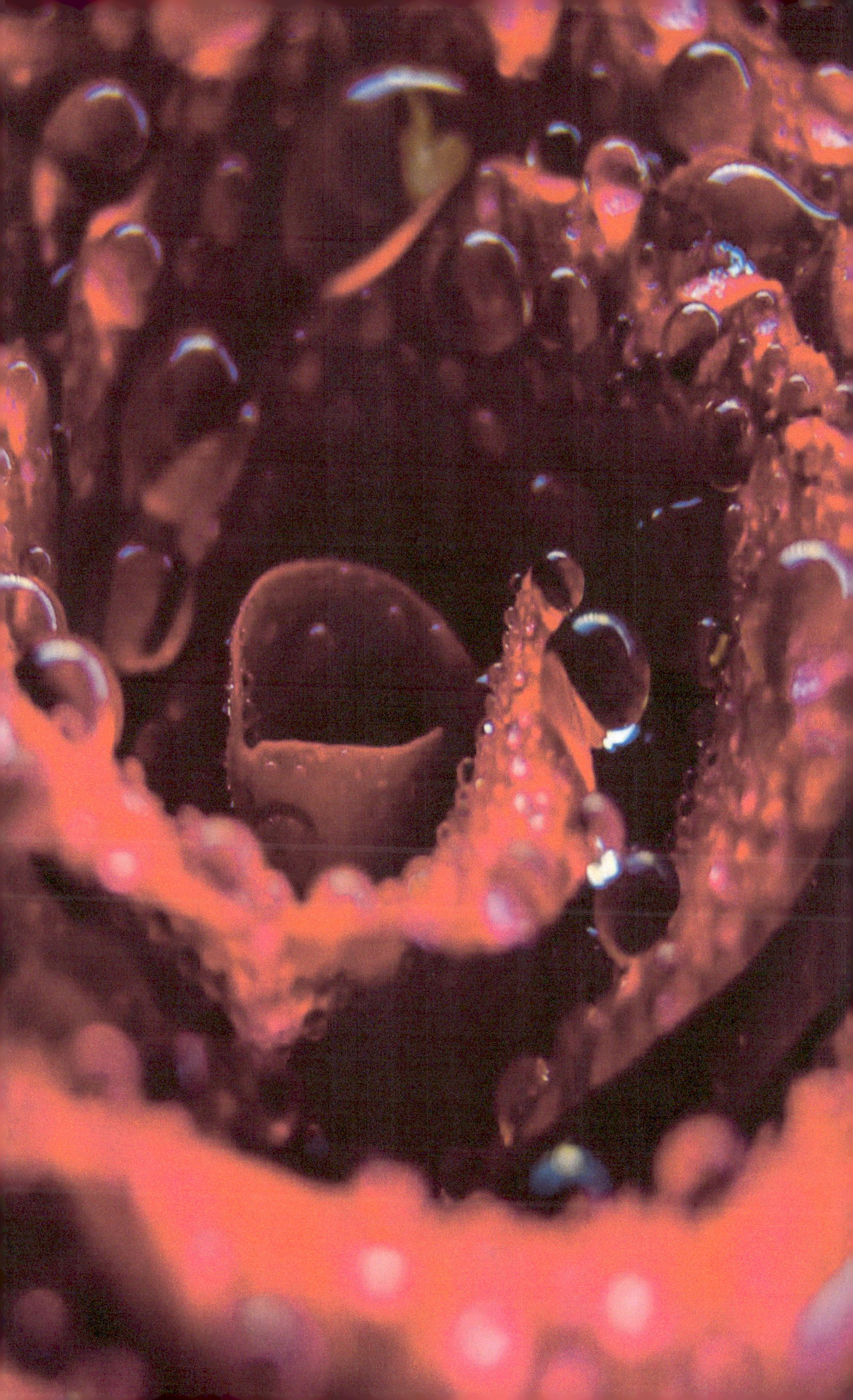

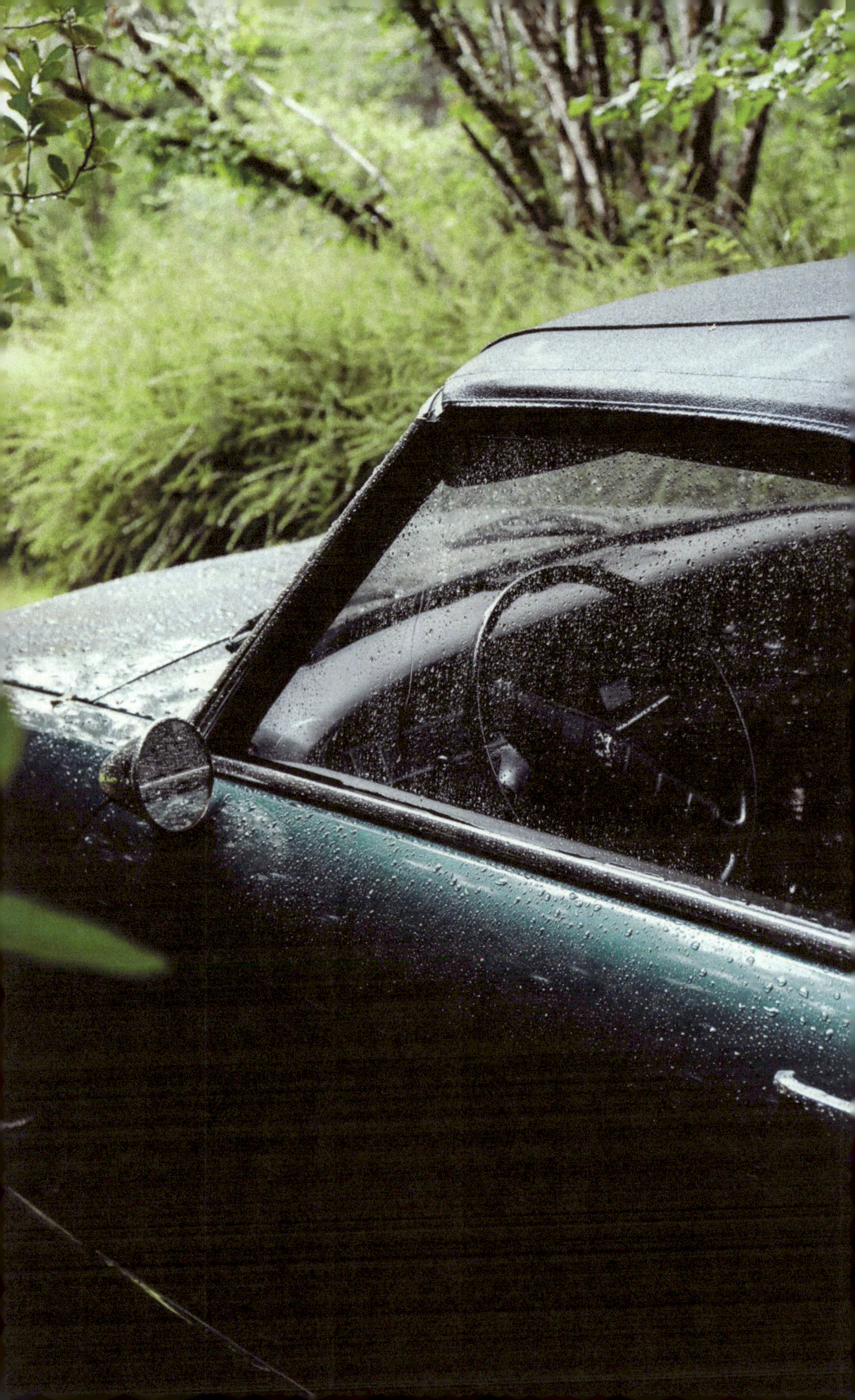

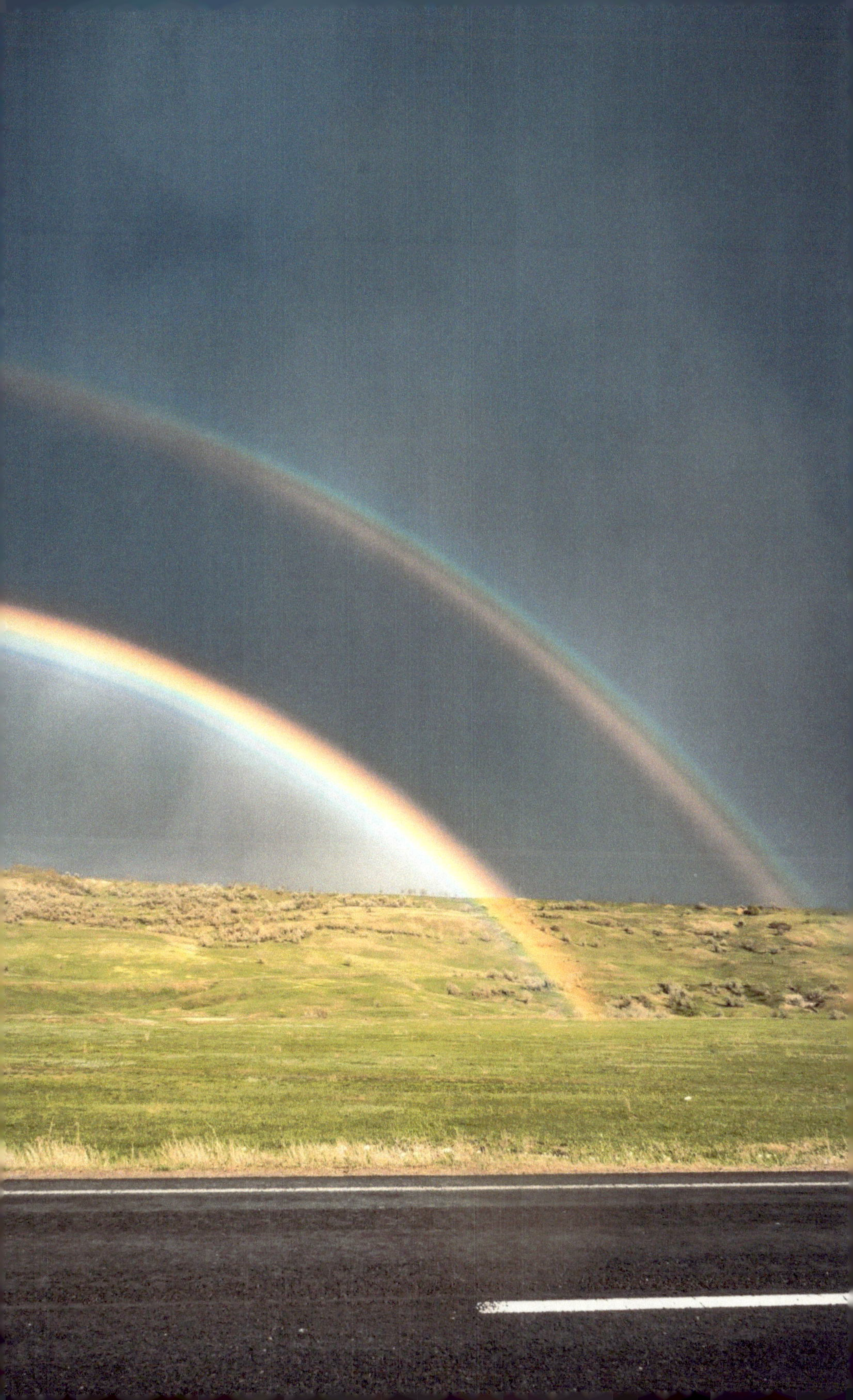

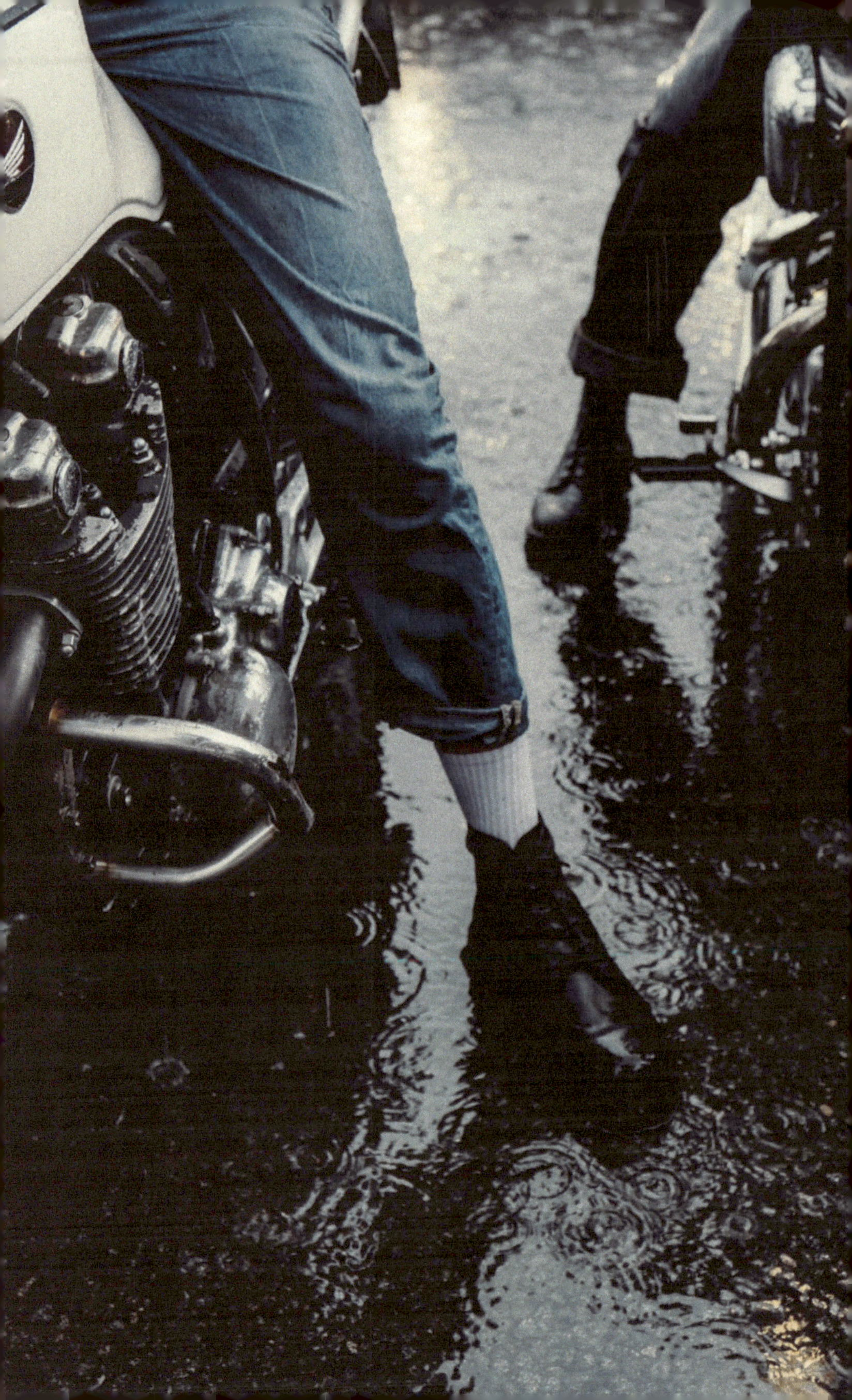

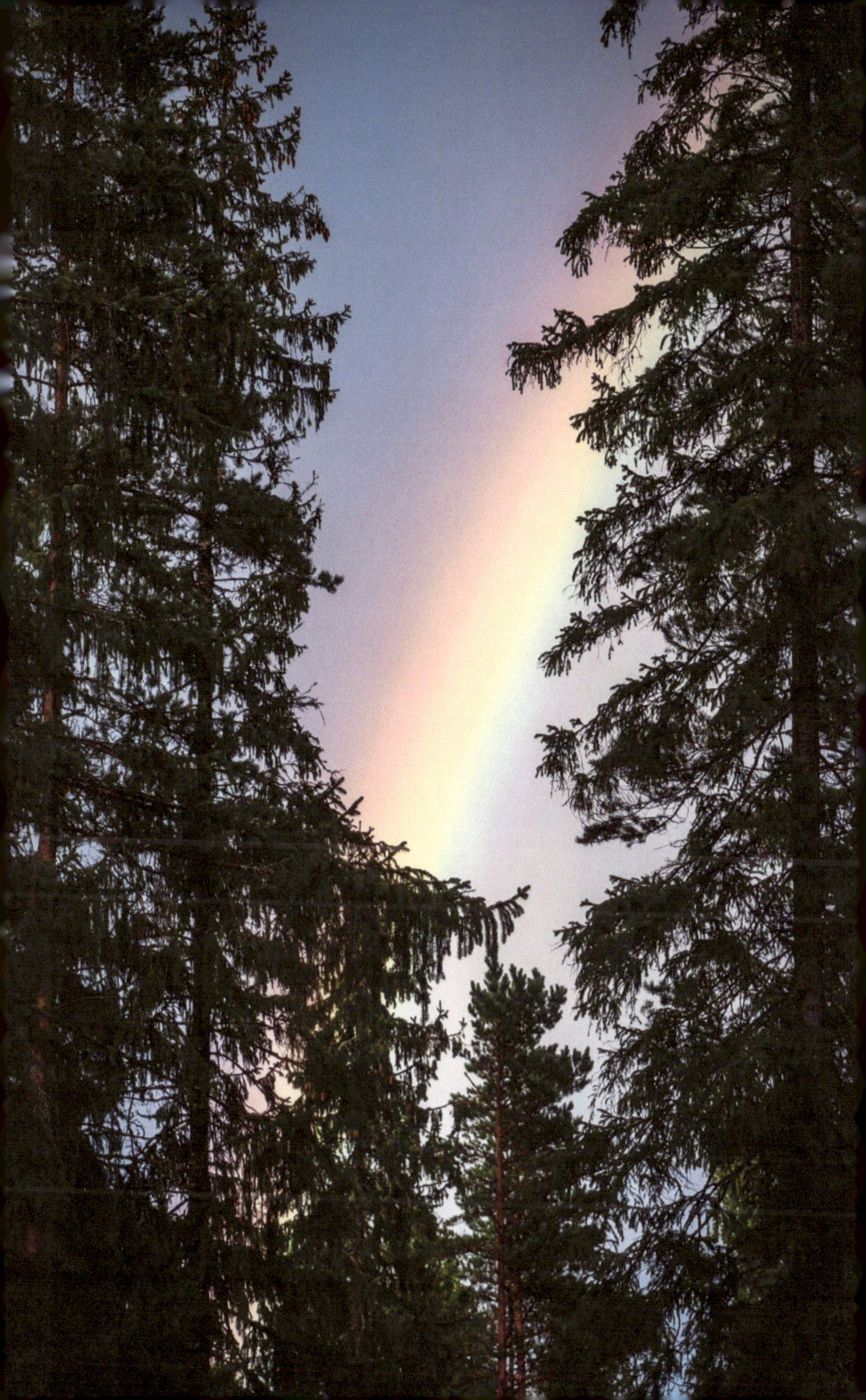

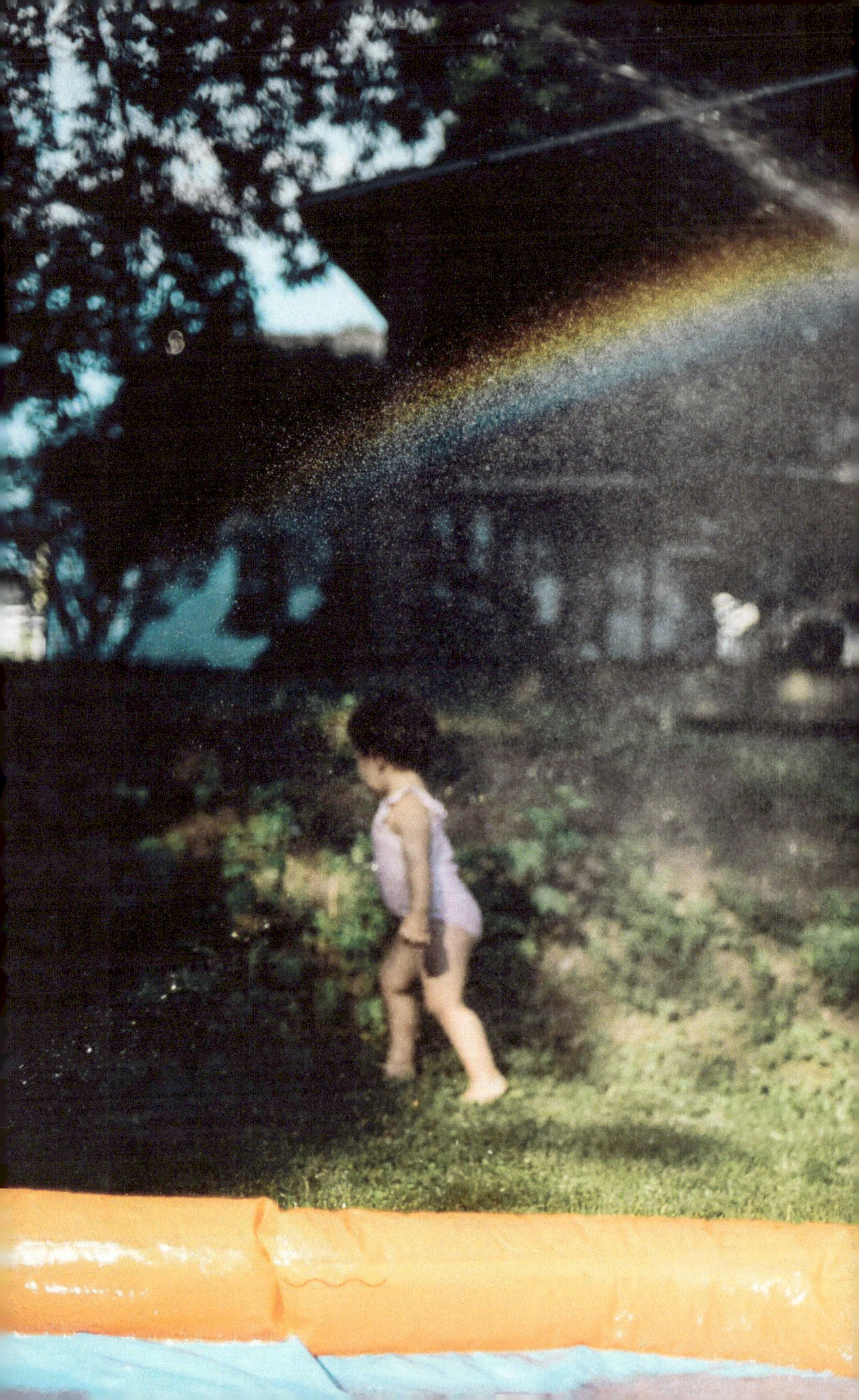

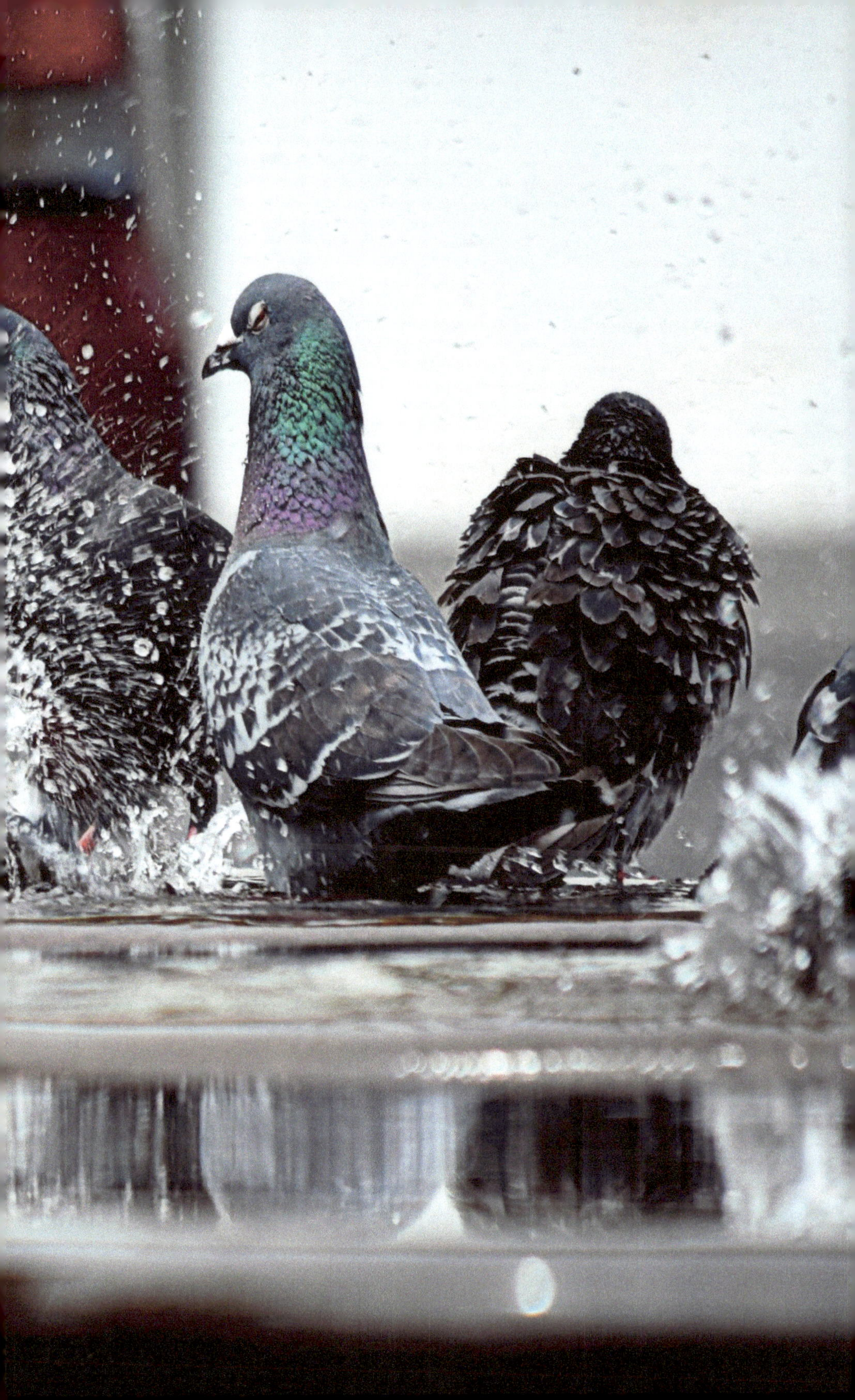

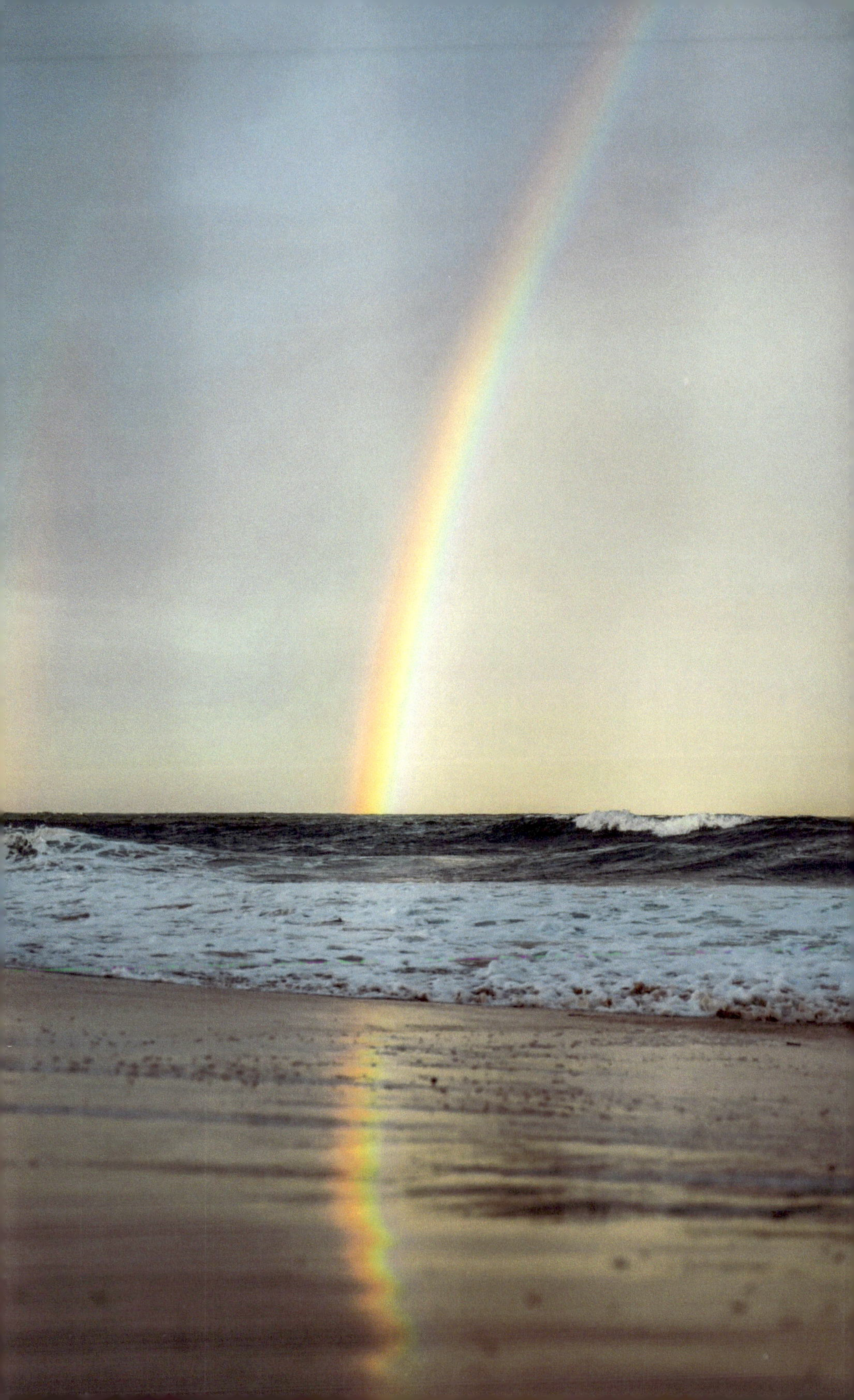

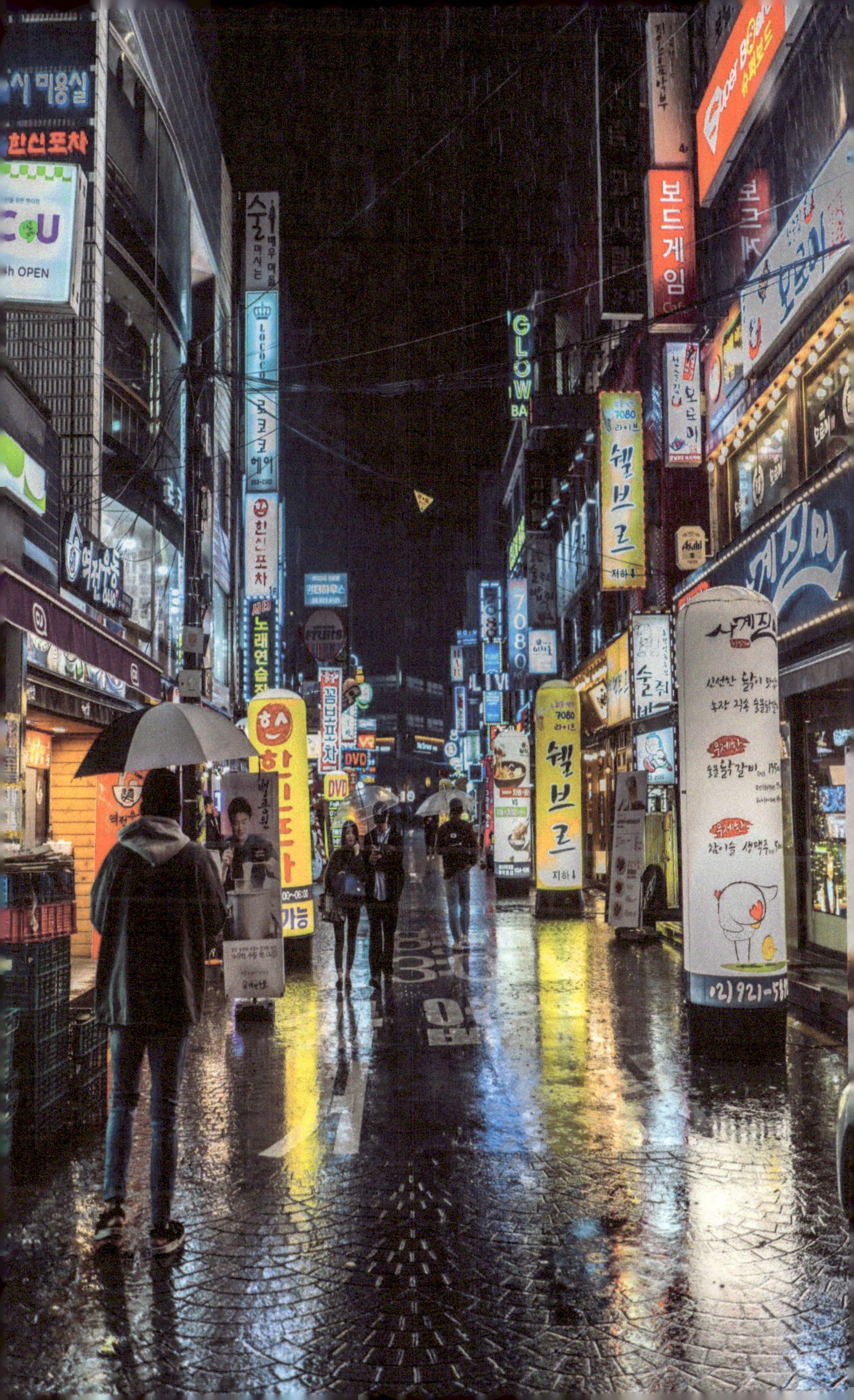

시 미용실
한신포차
CU
h OPEN
보드게임
GLOW
7080
라이브
쉘브르
지하
로코코헤어
LOCOCO
한신포차
노래연습장
DVD

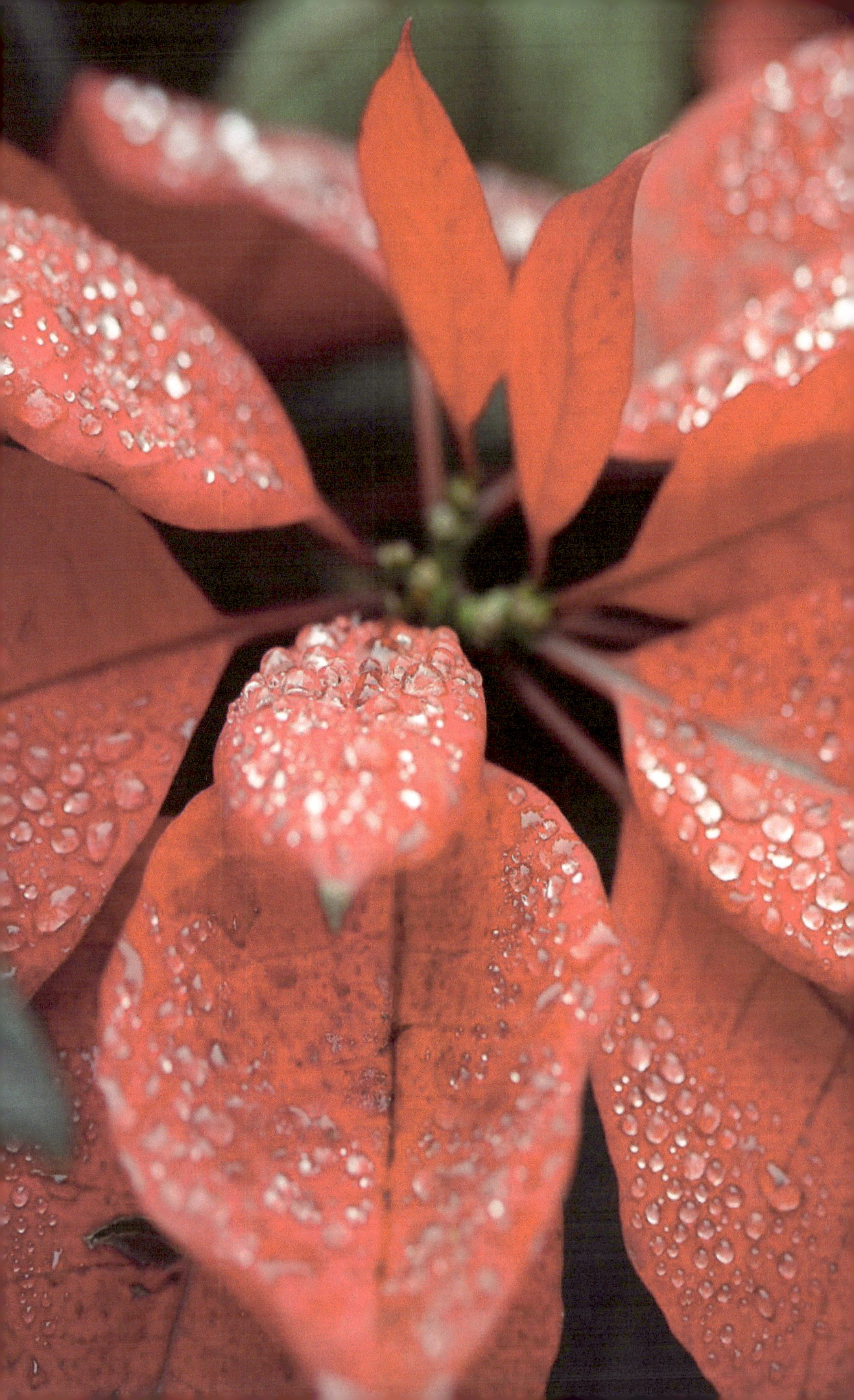

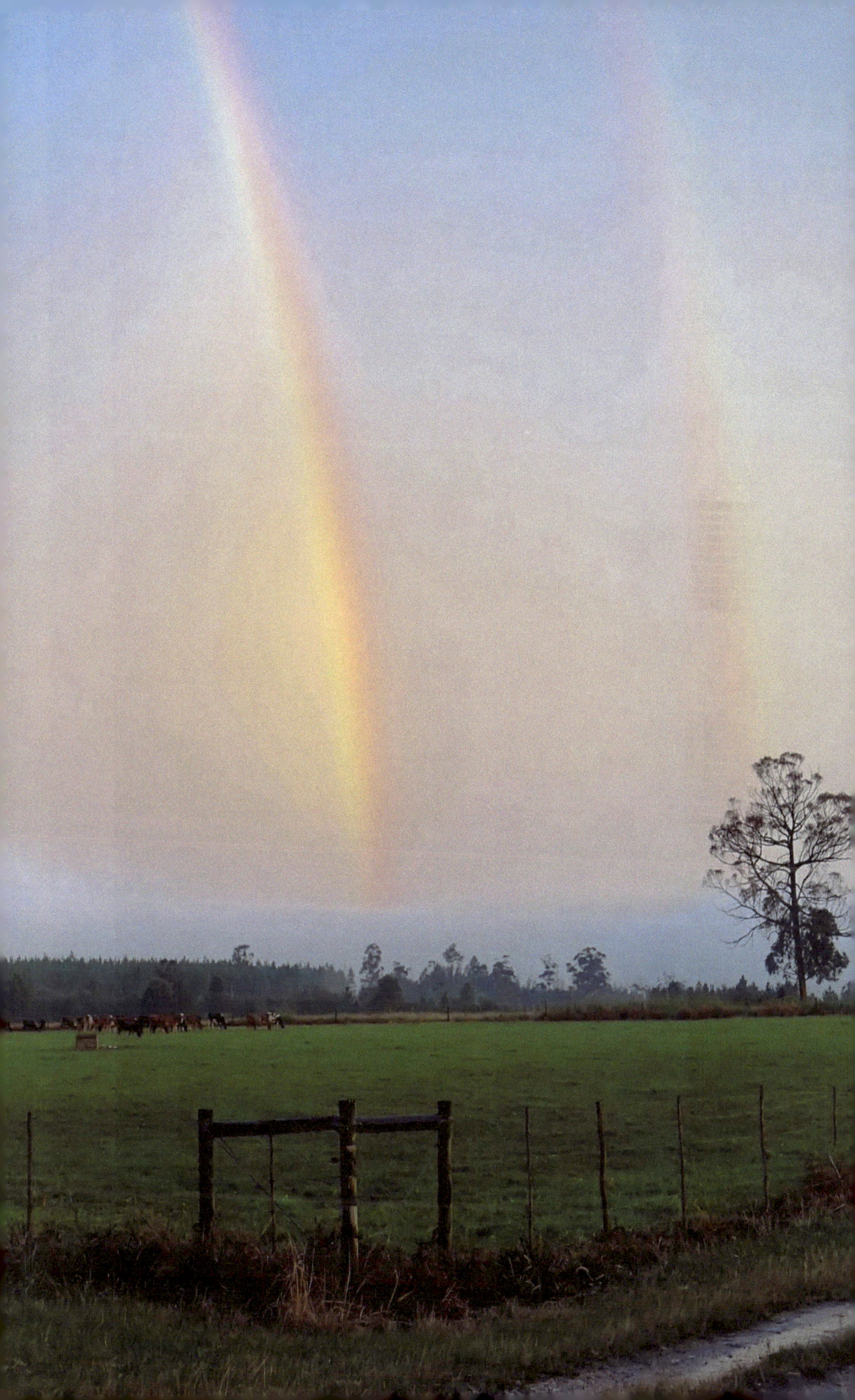

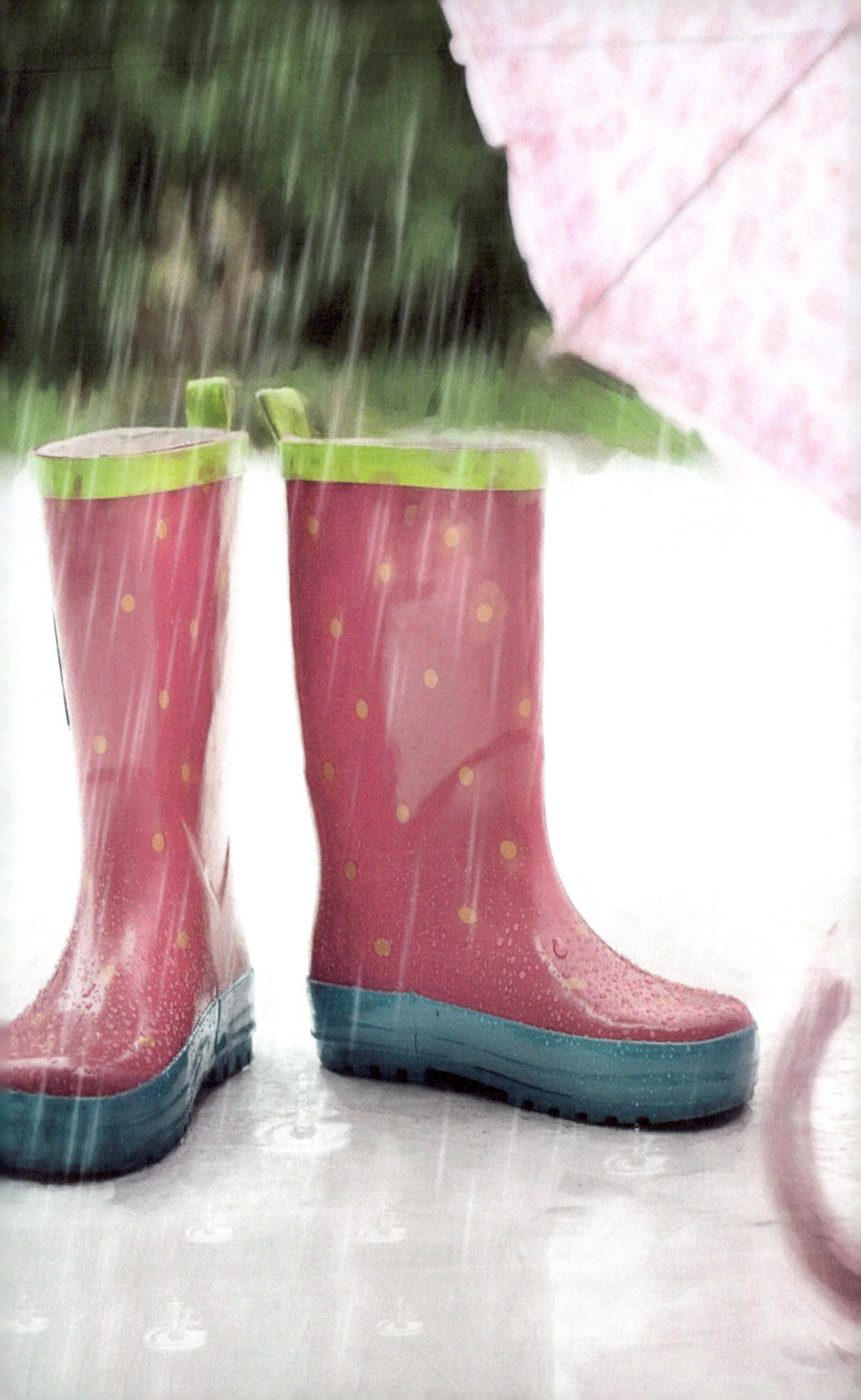

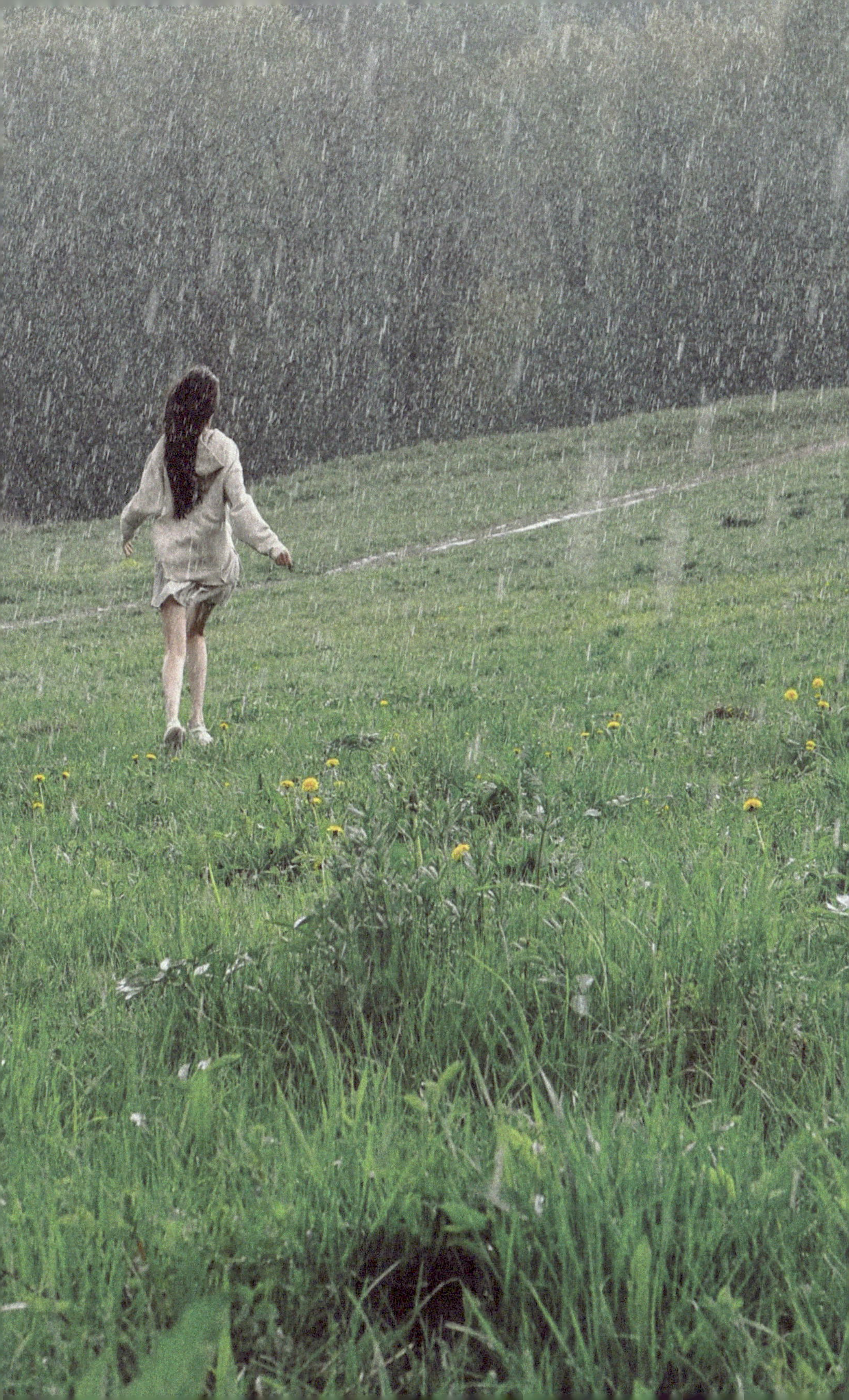

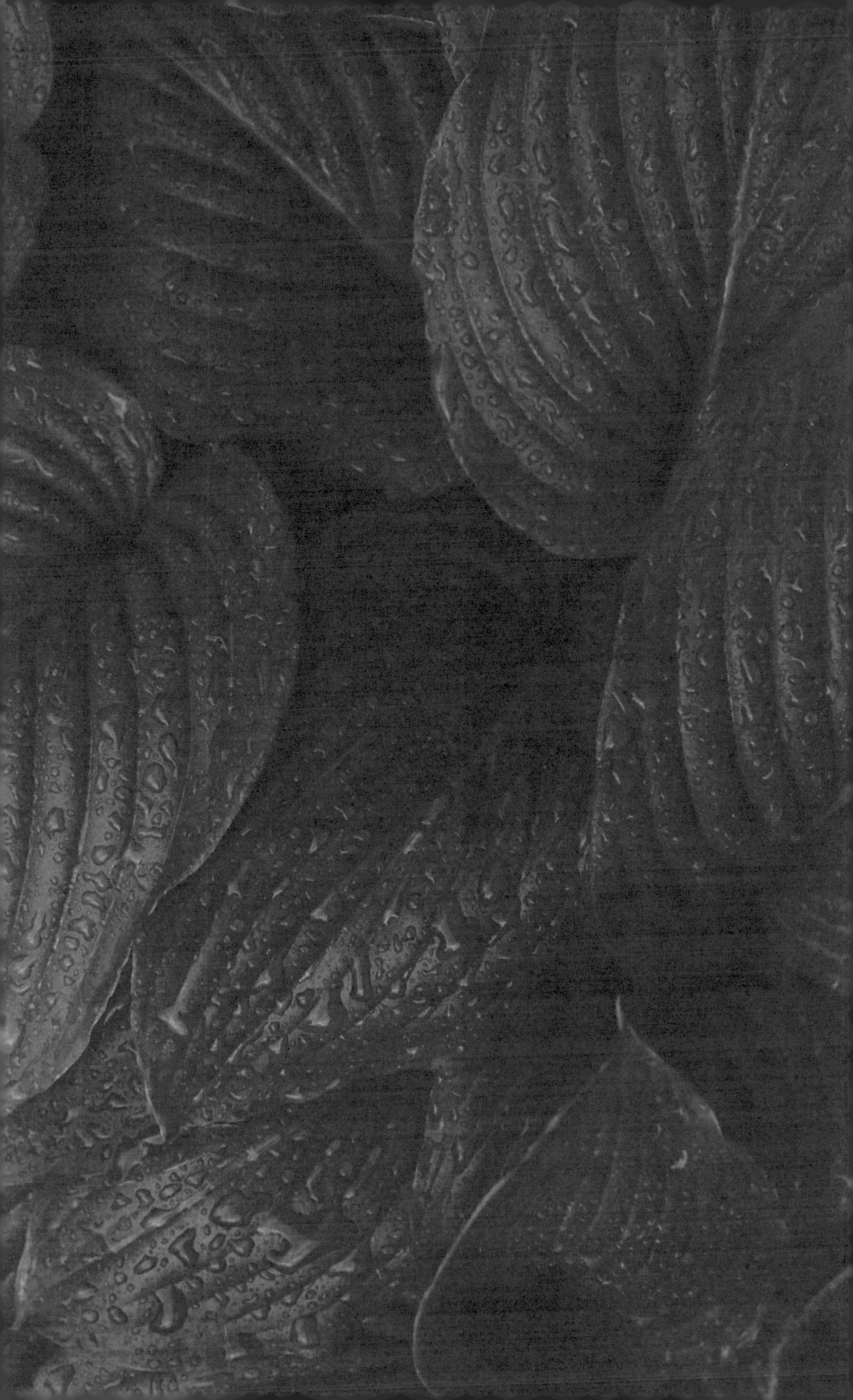

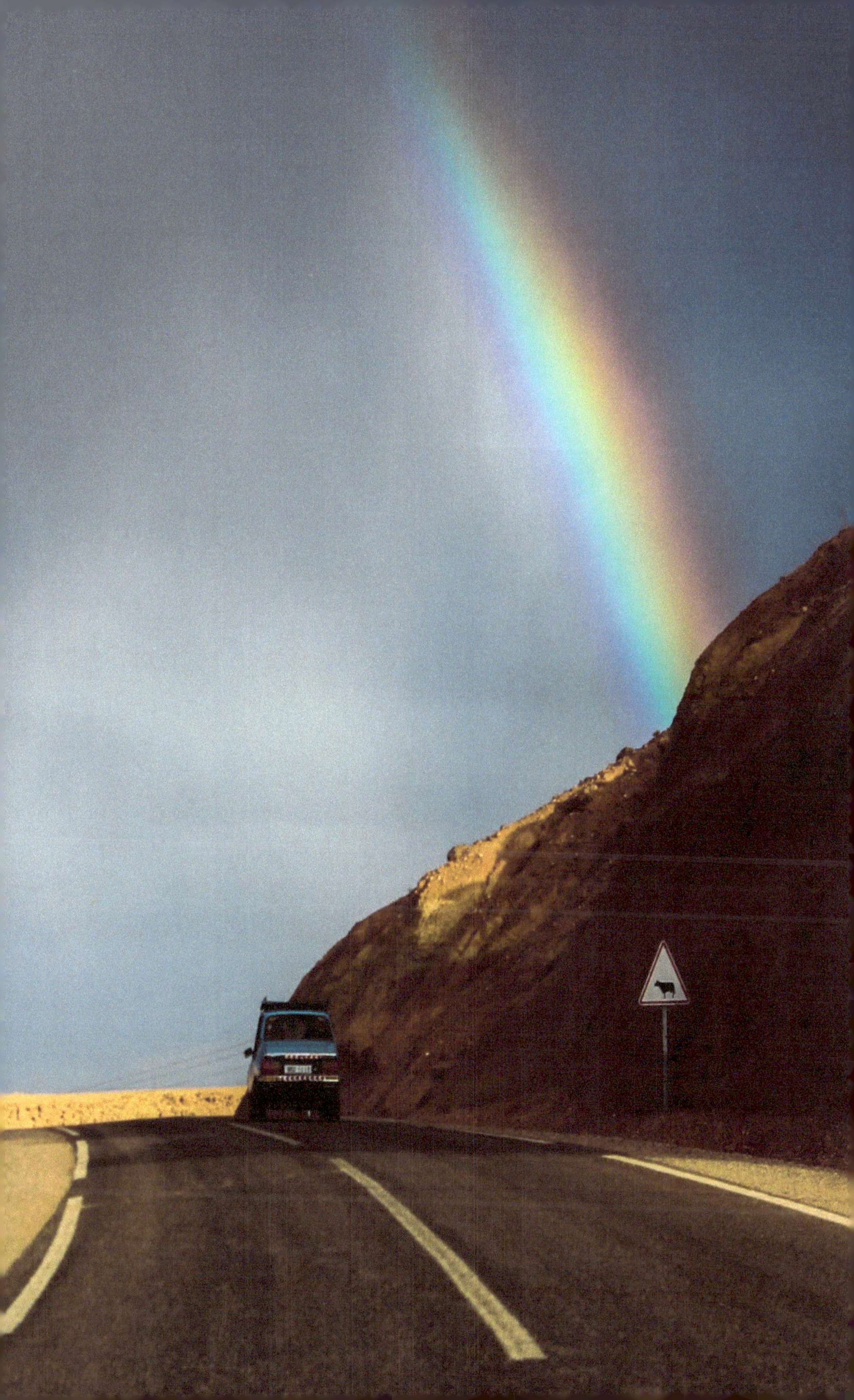

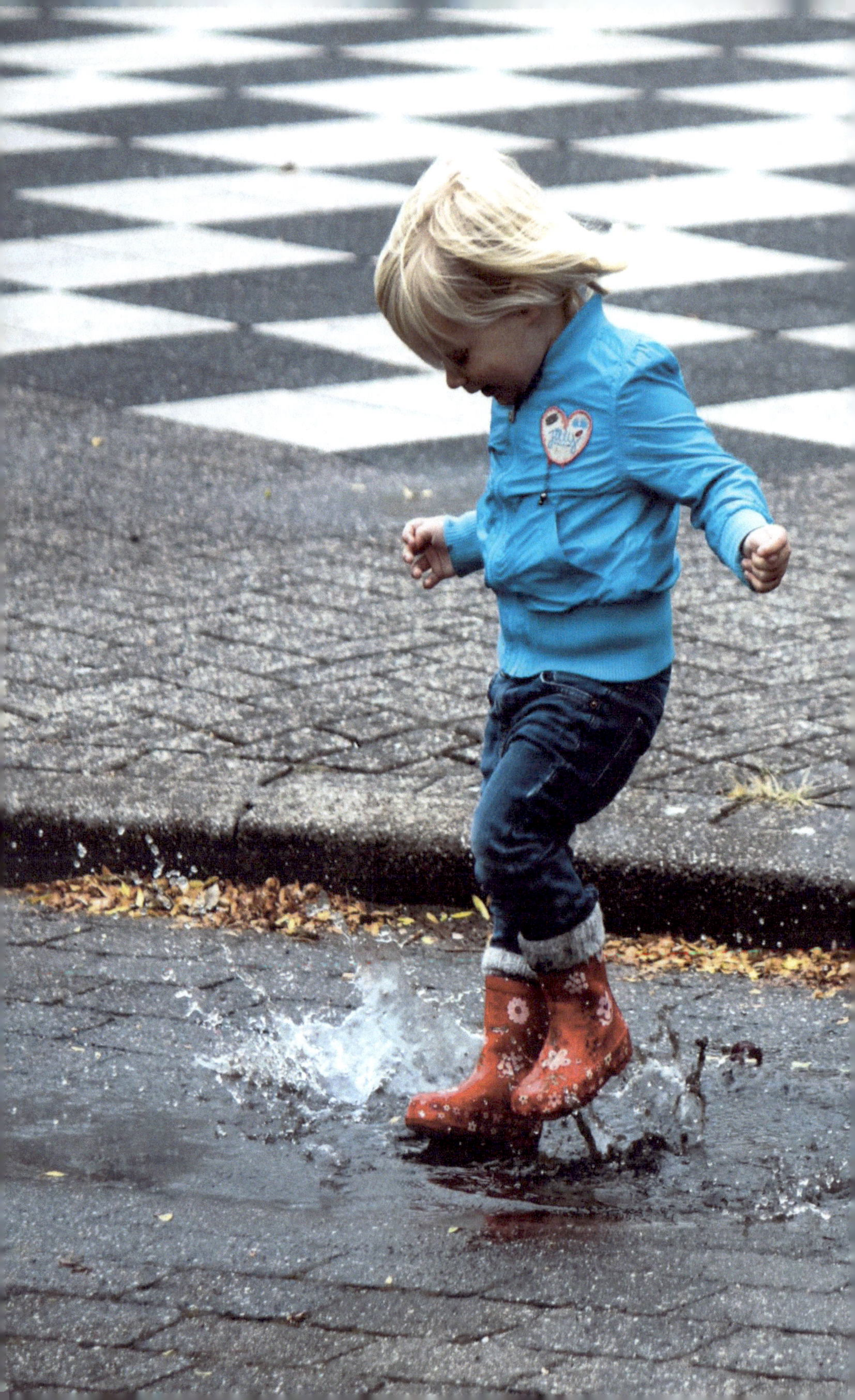

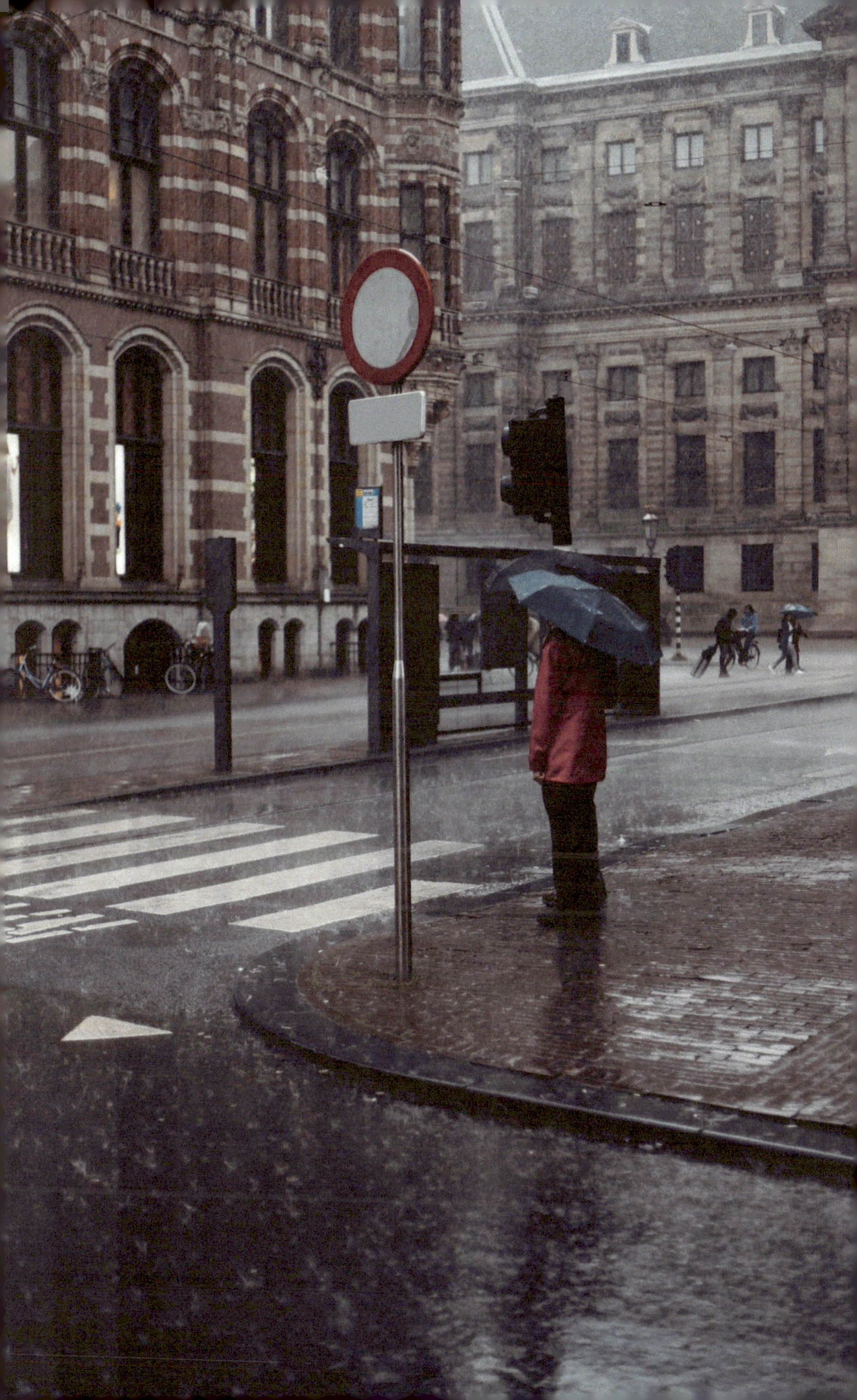

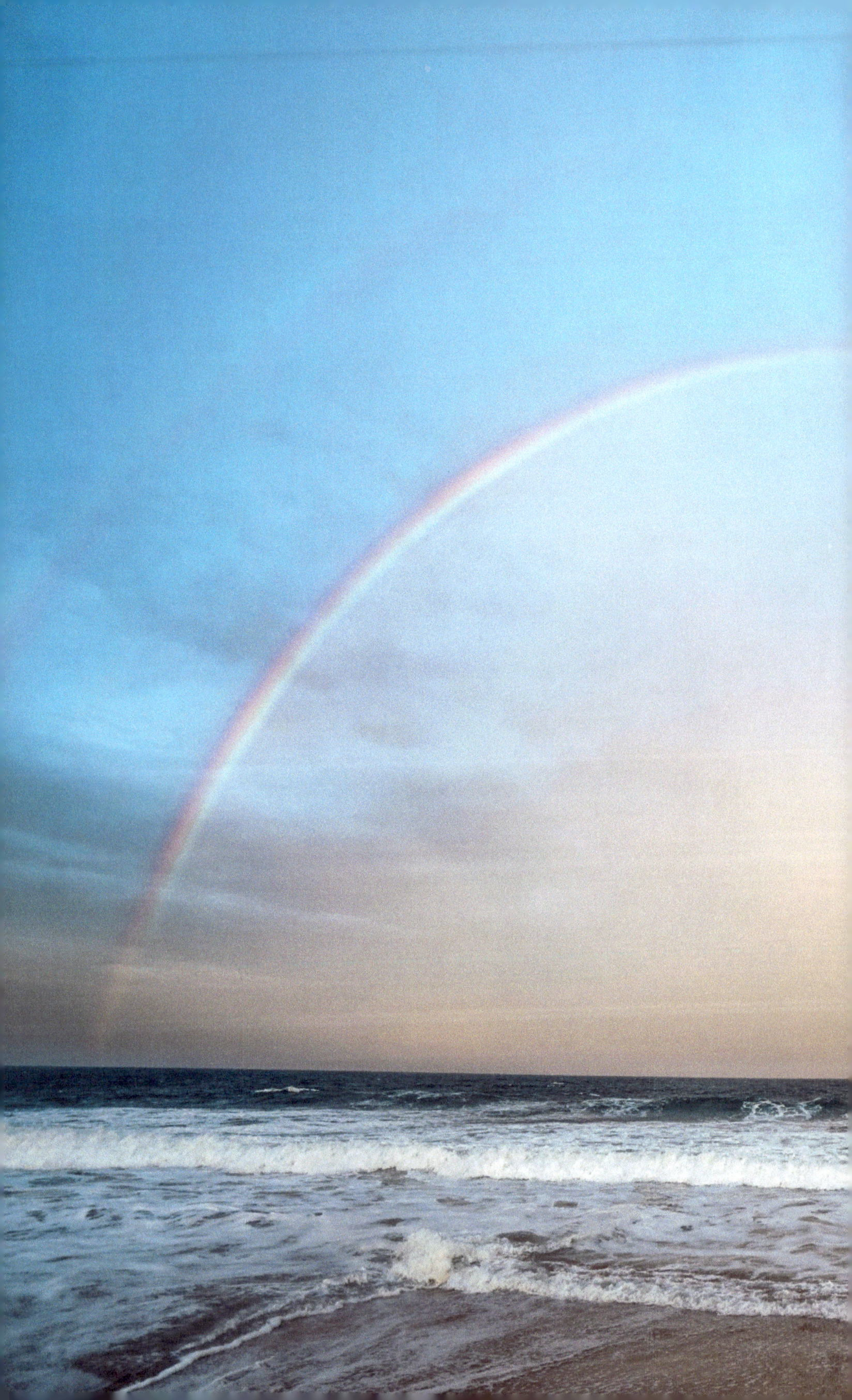

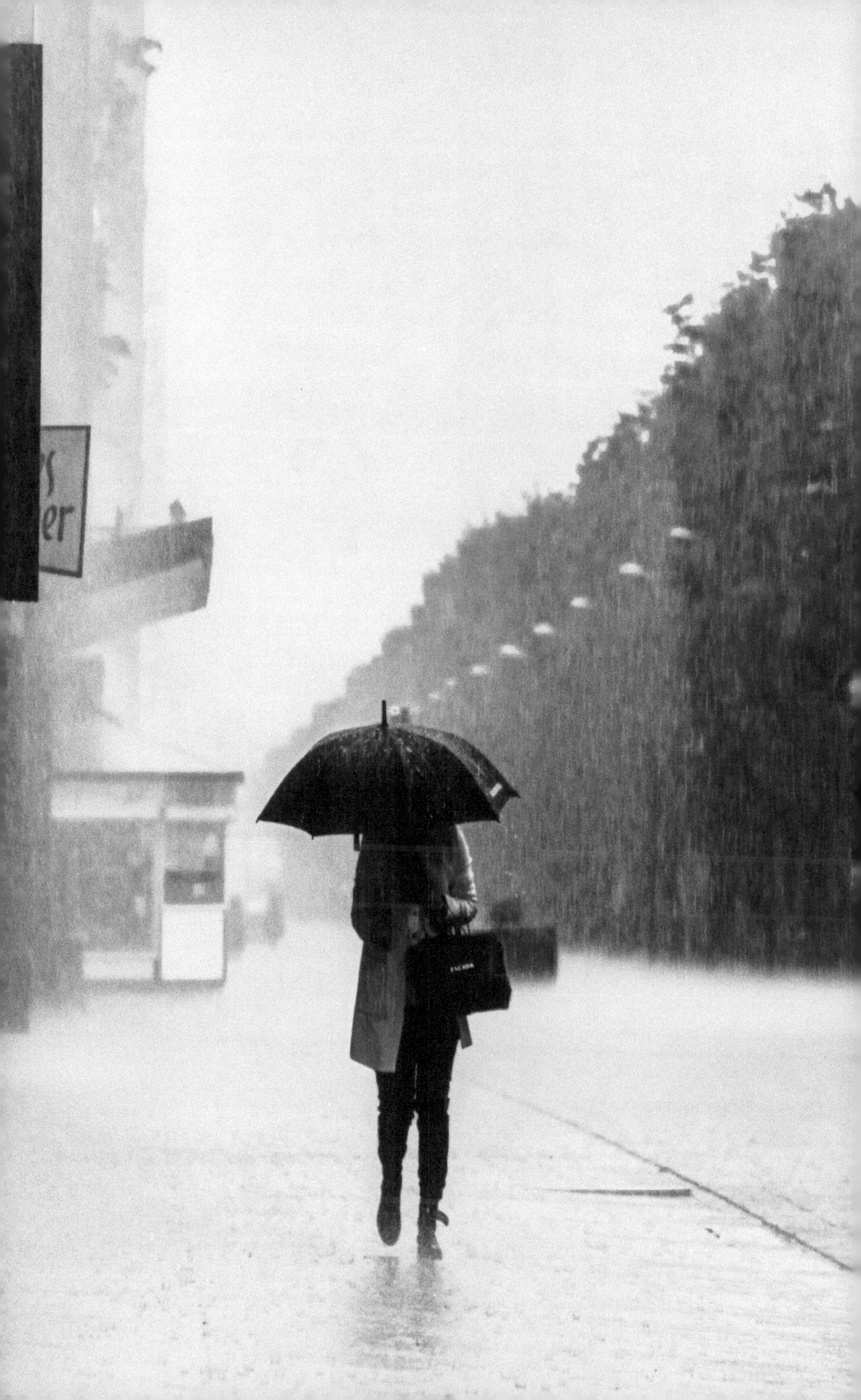

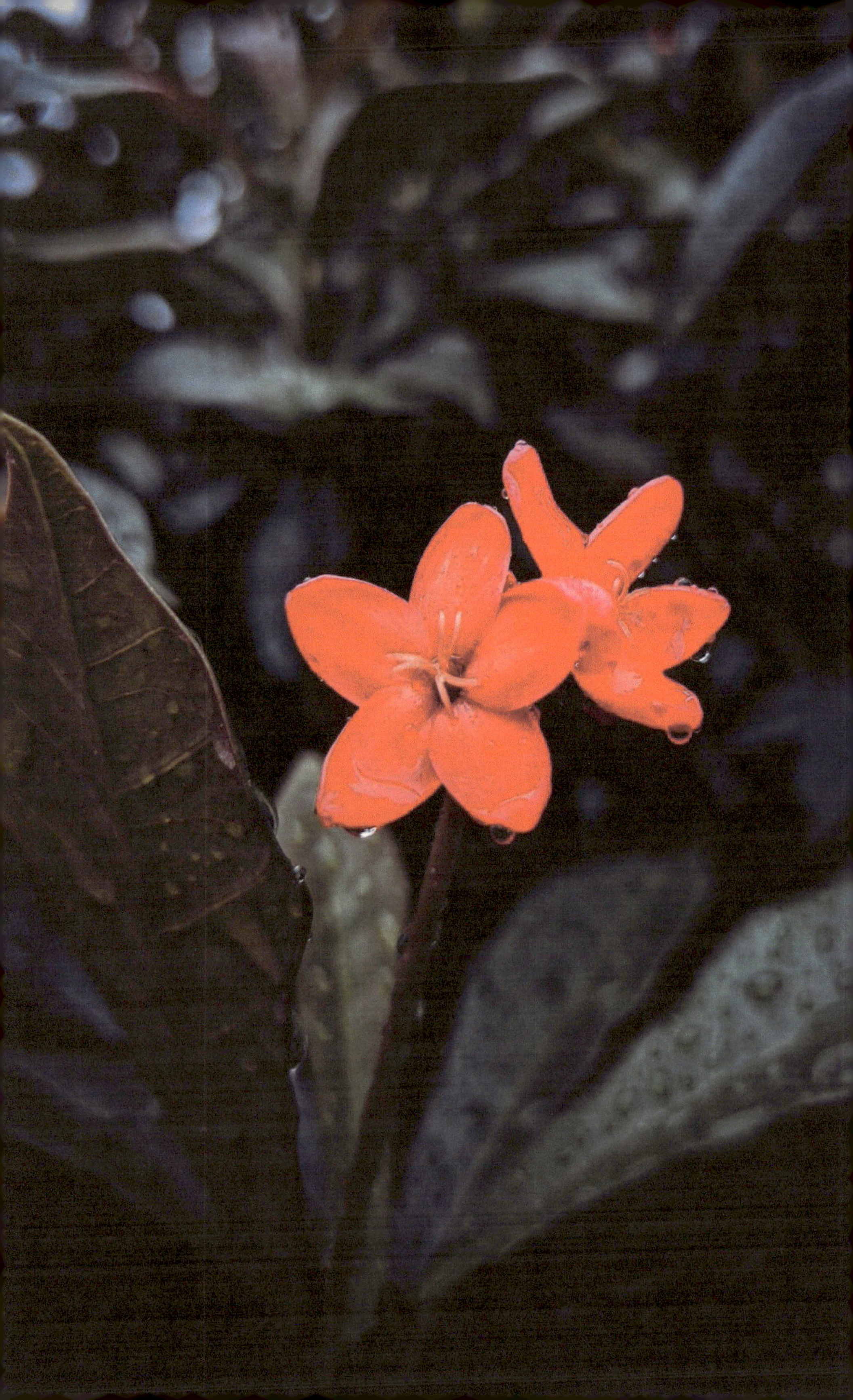

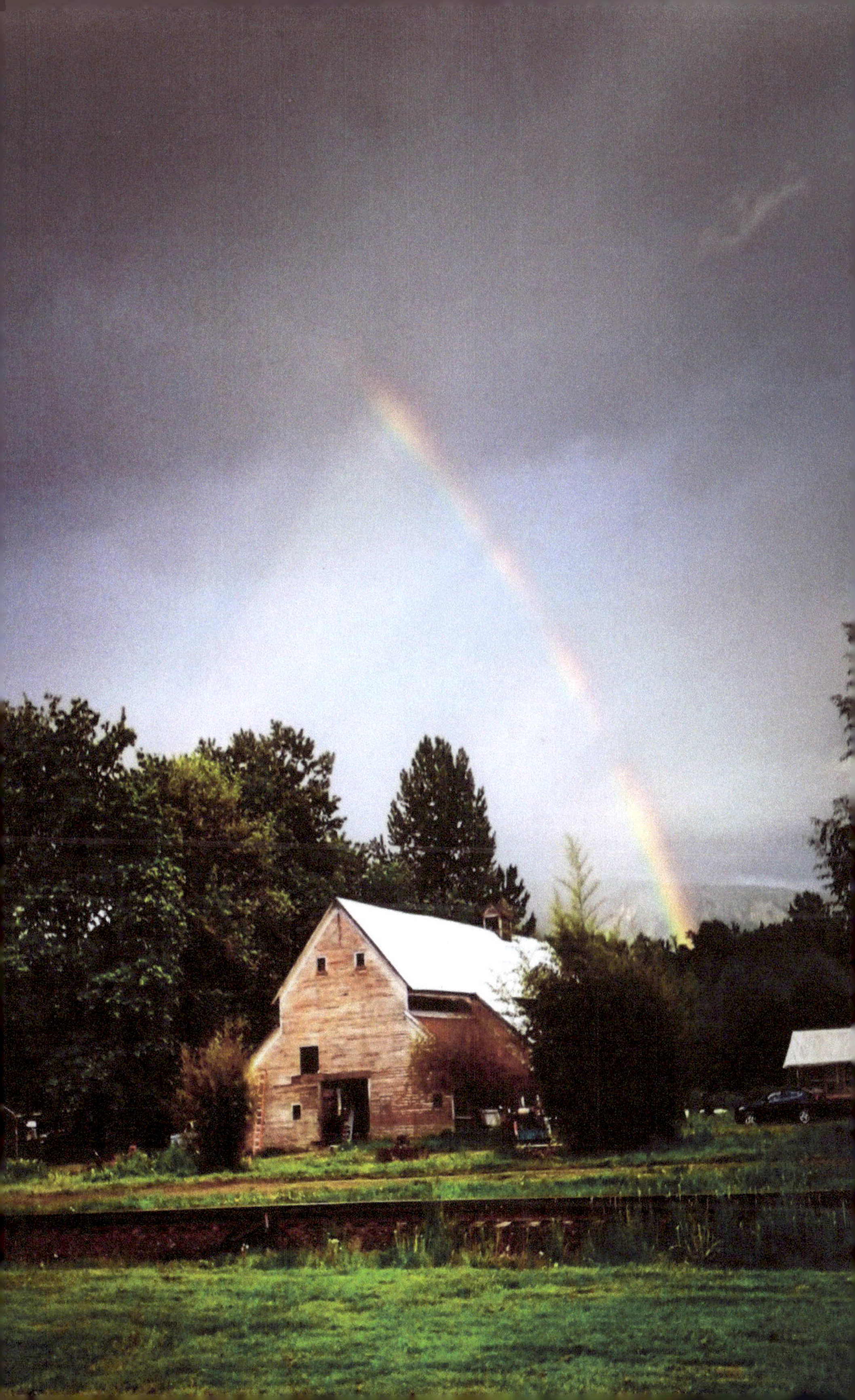

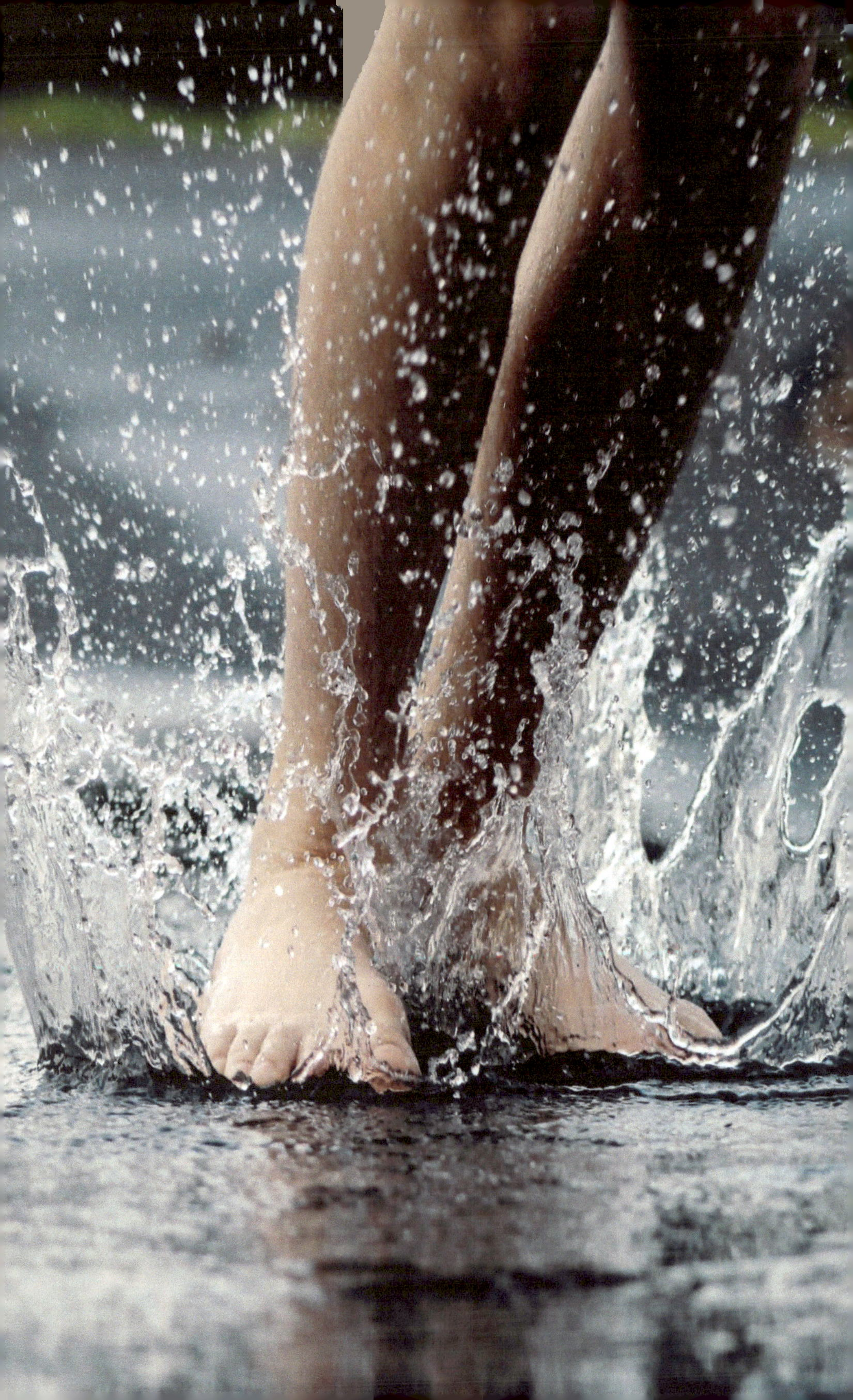

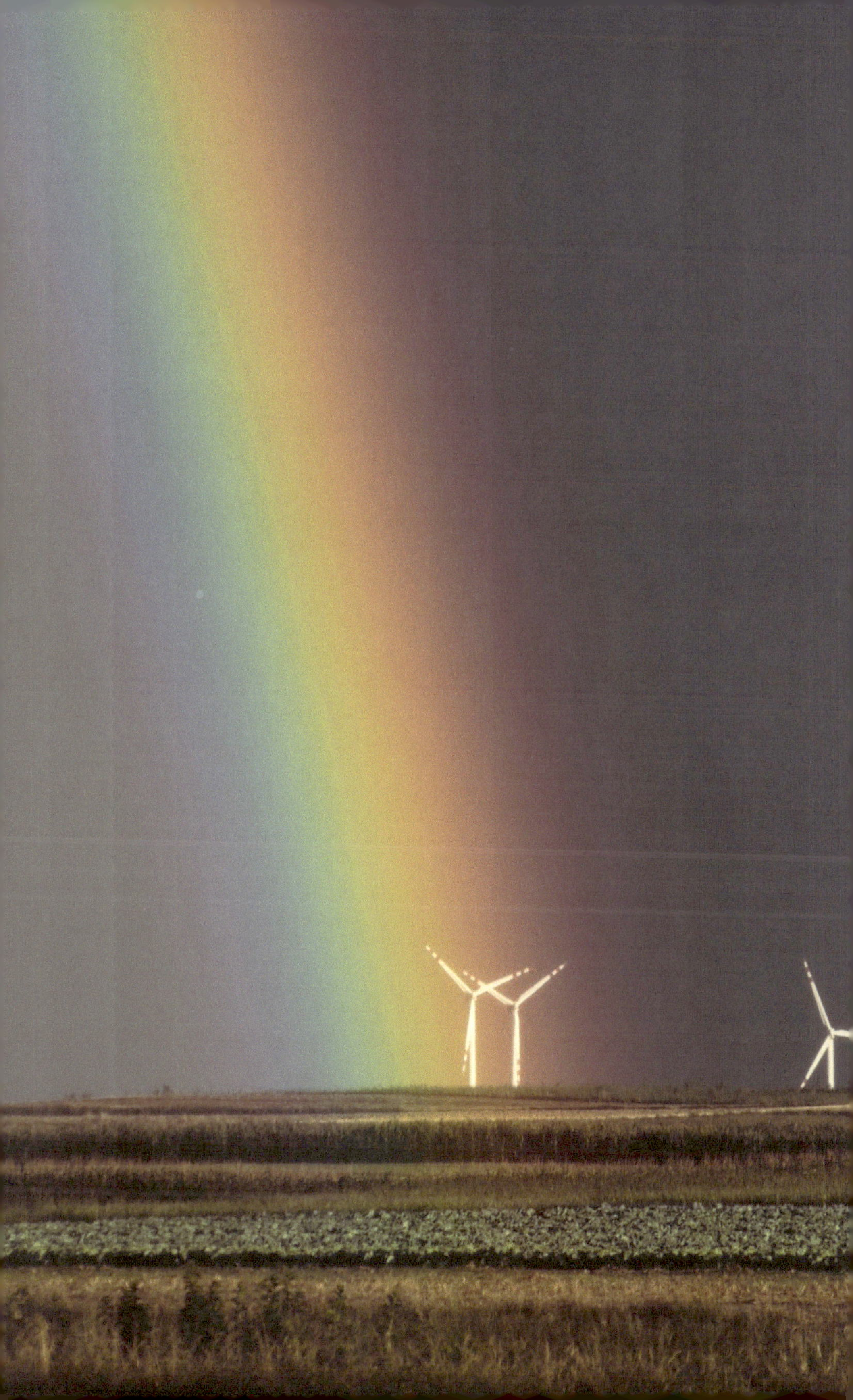

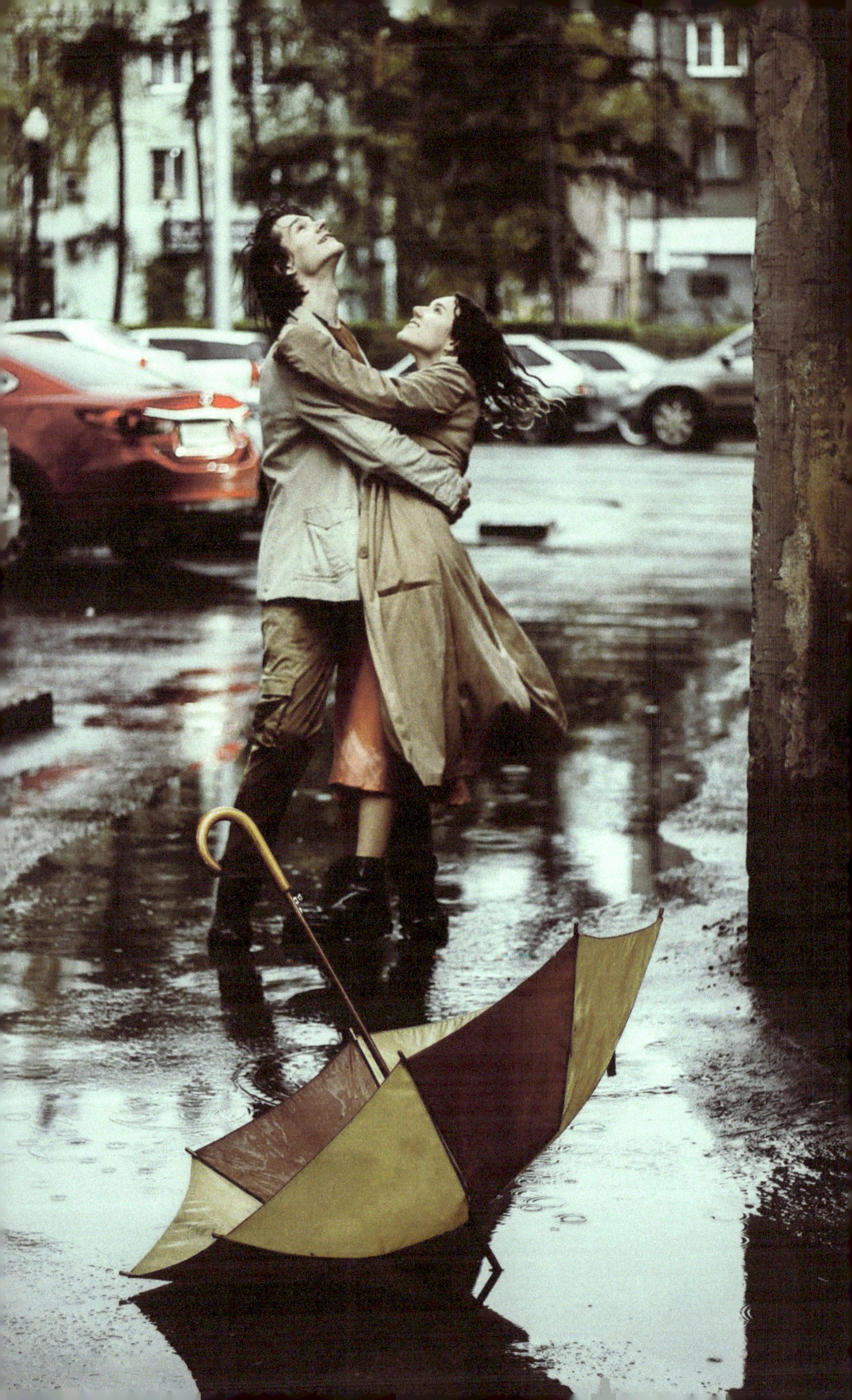

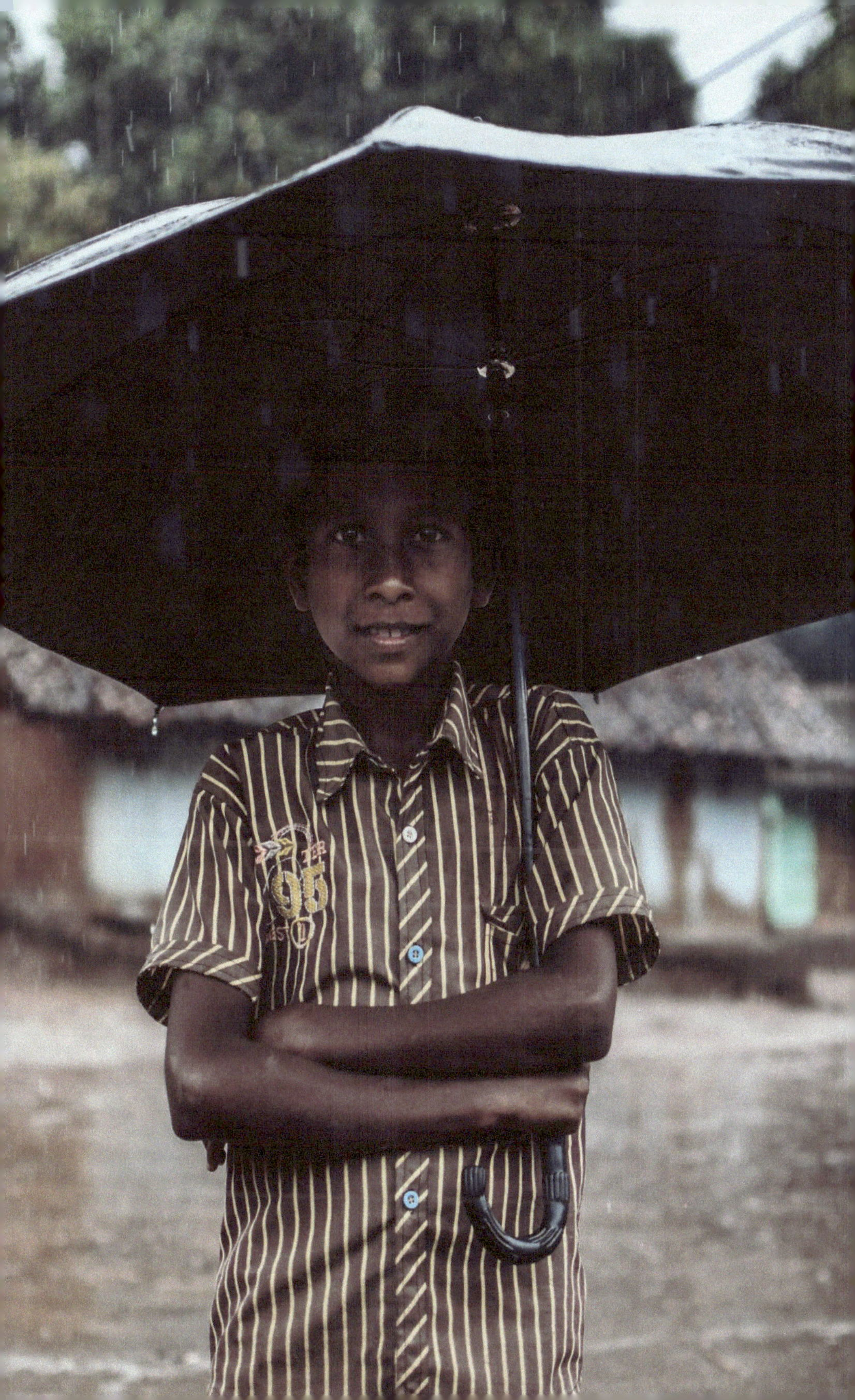
95

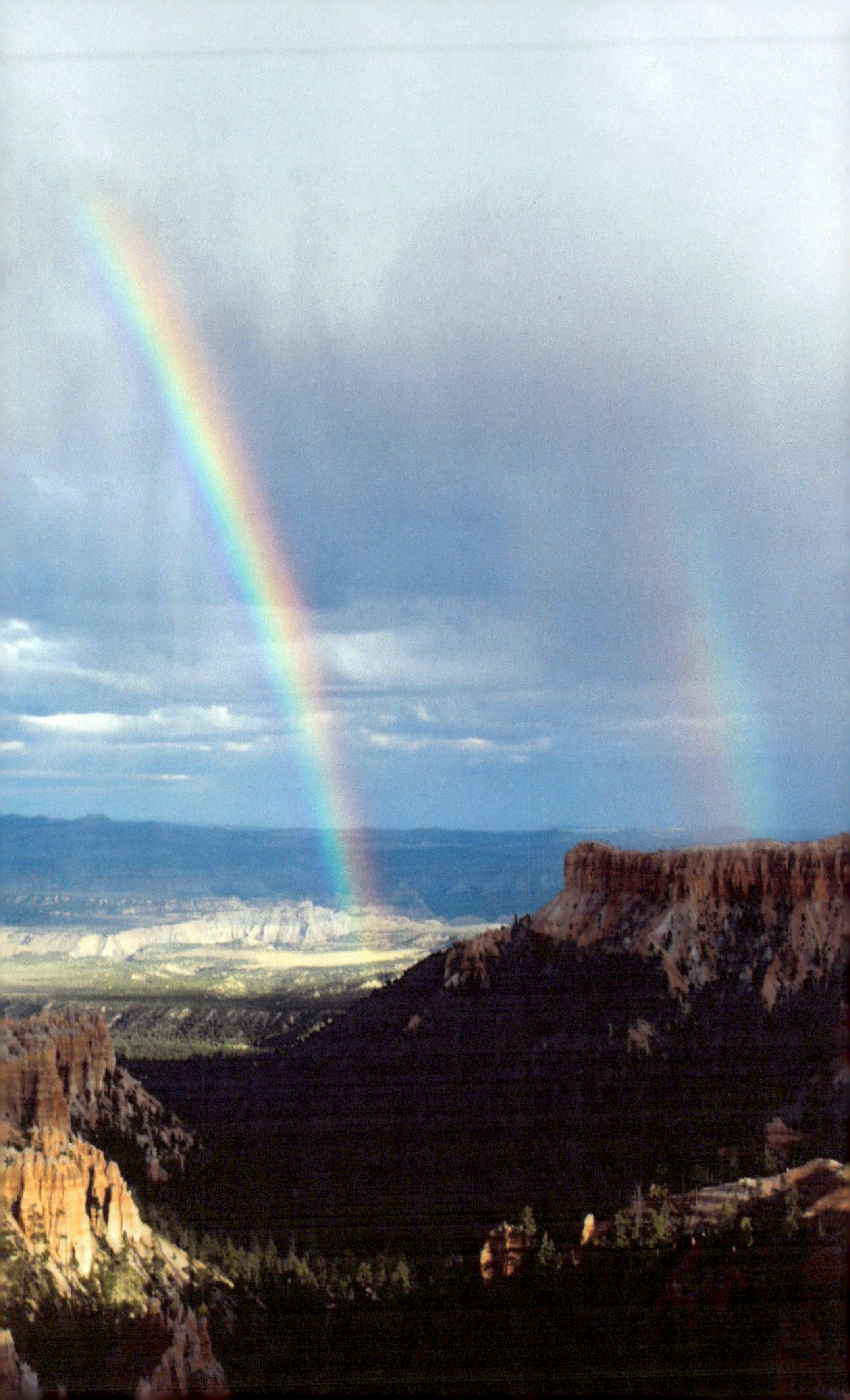

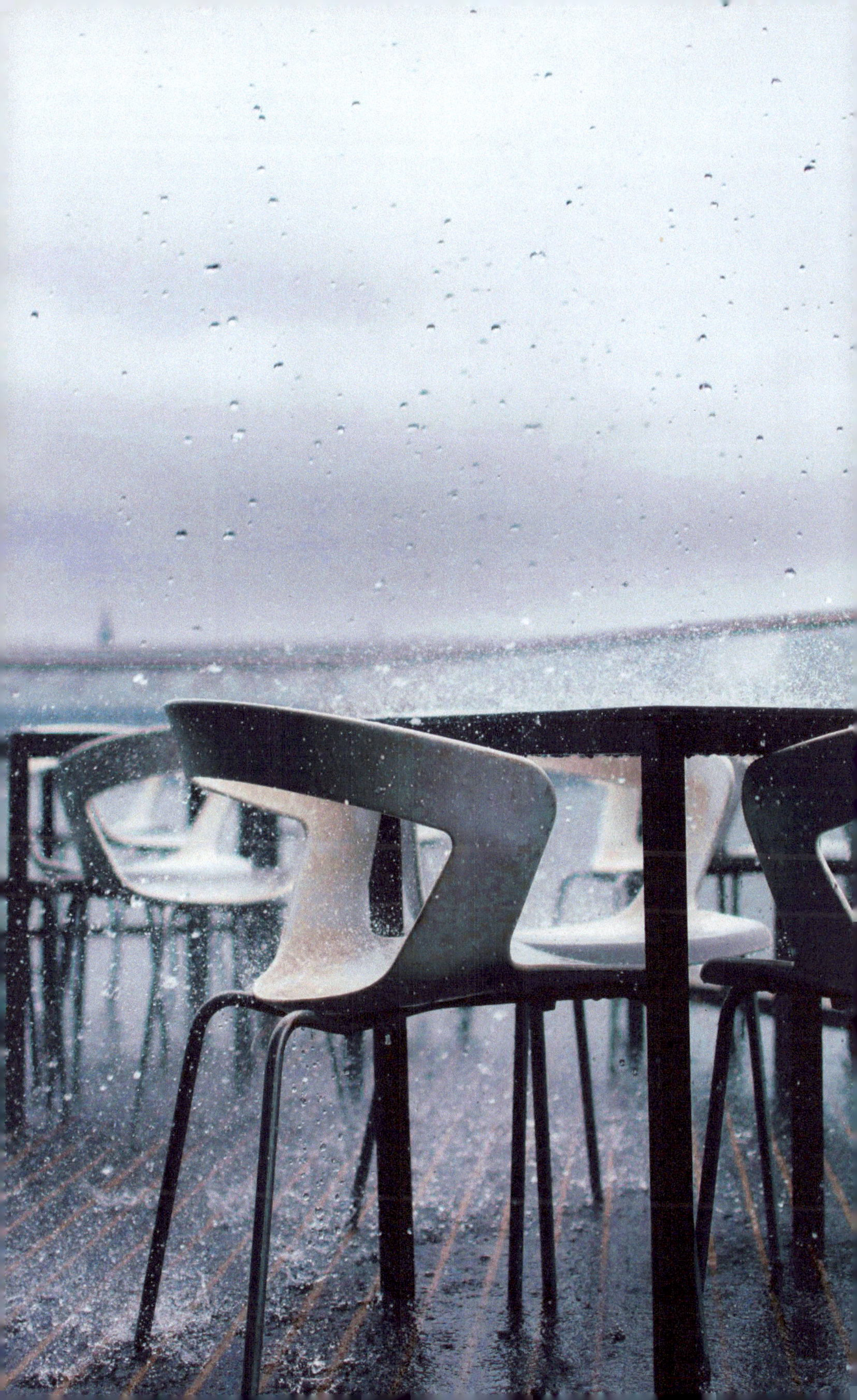

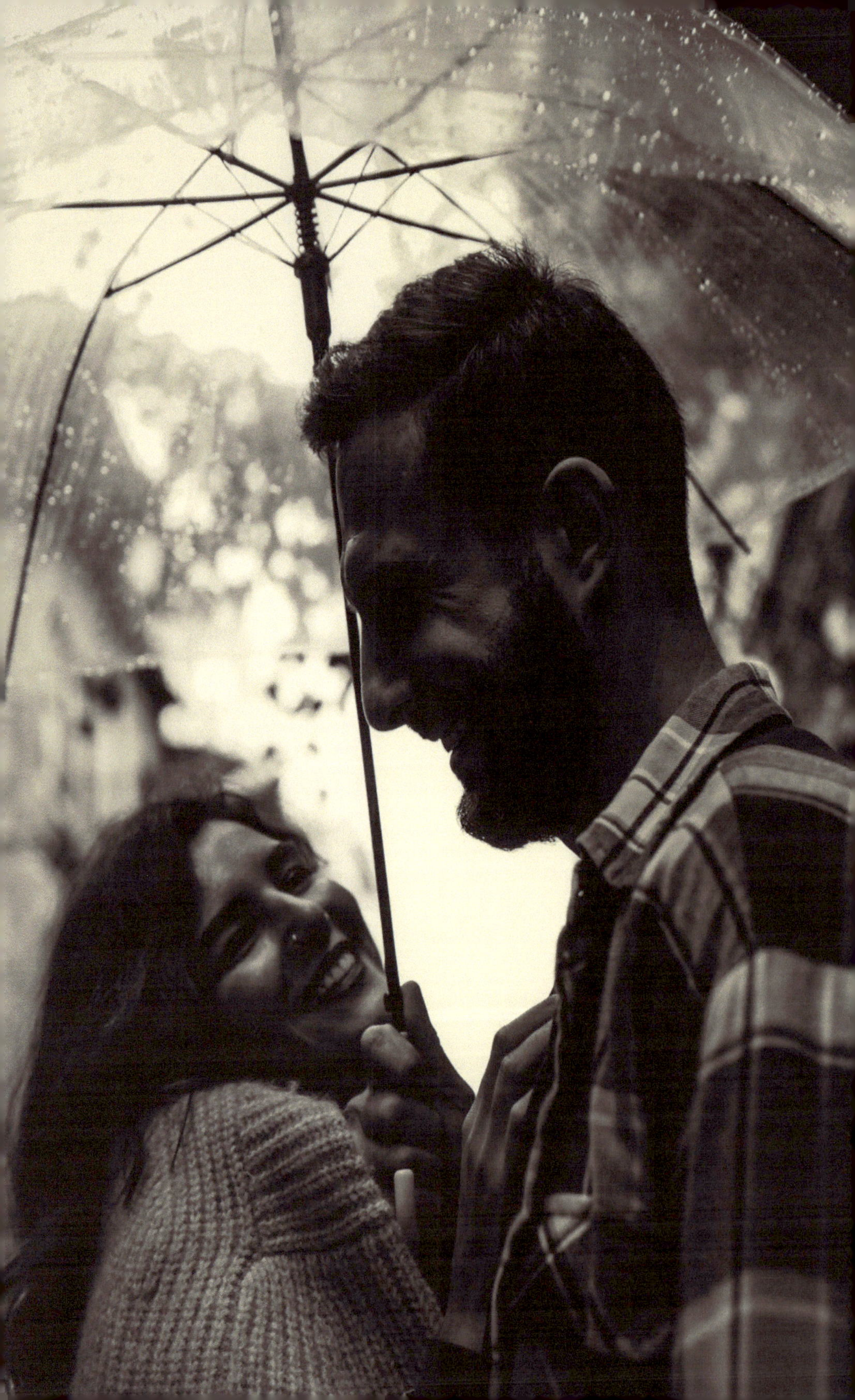

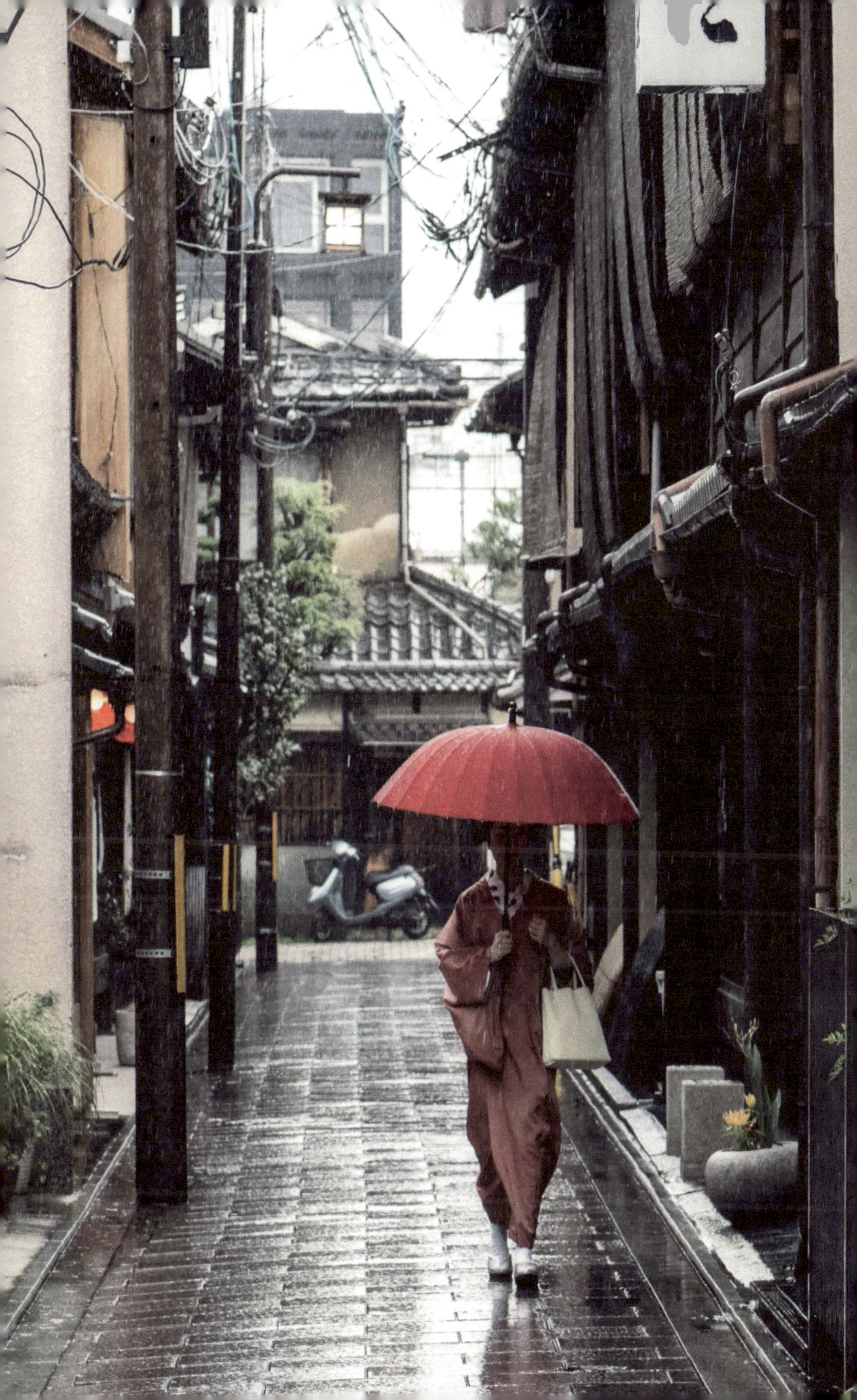

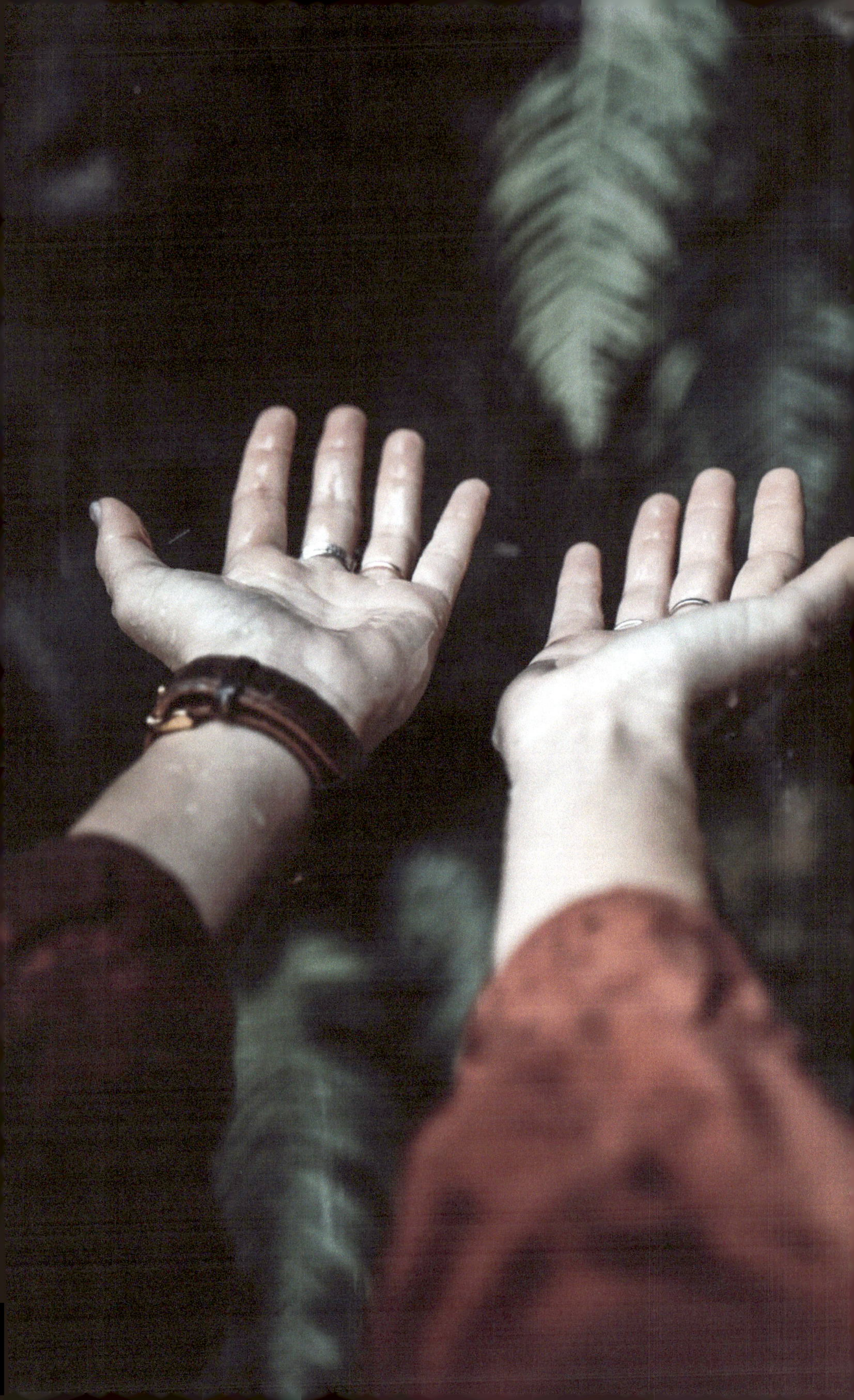

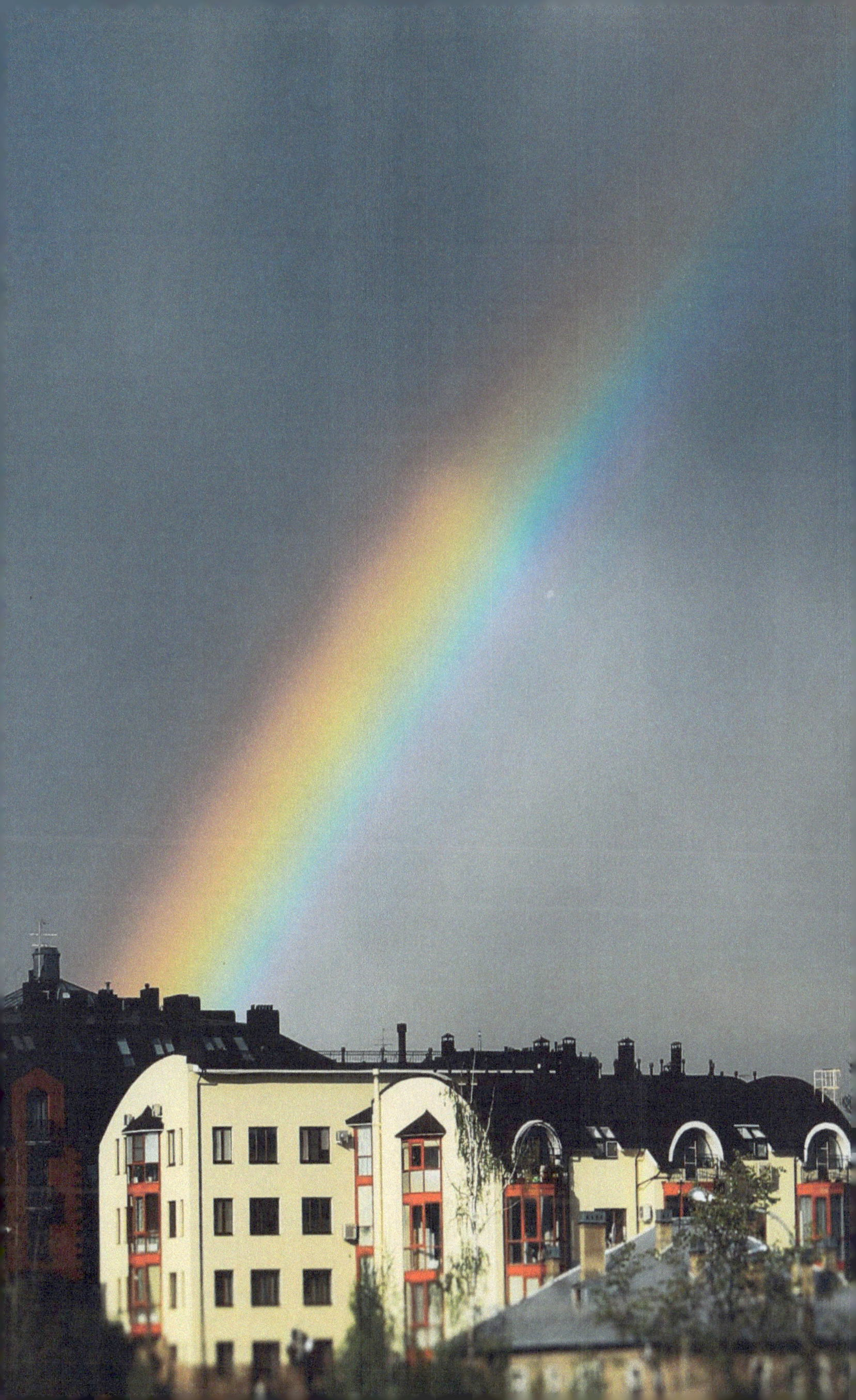

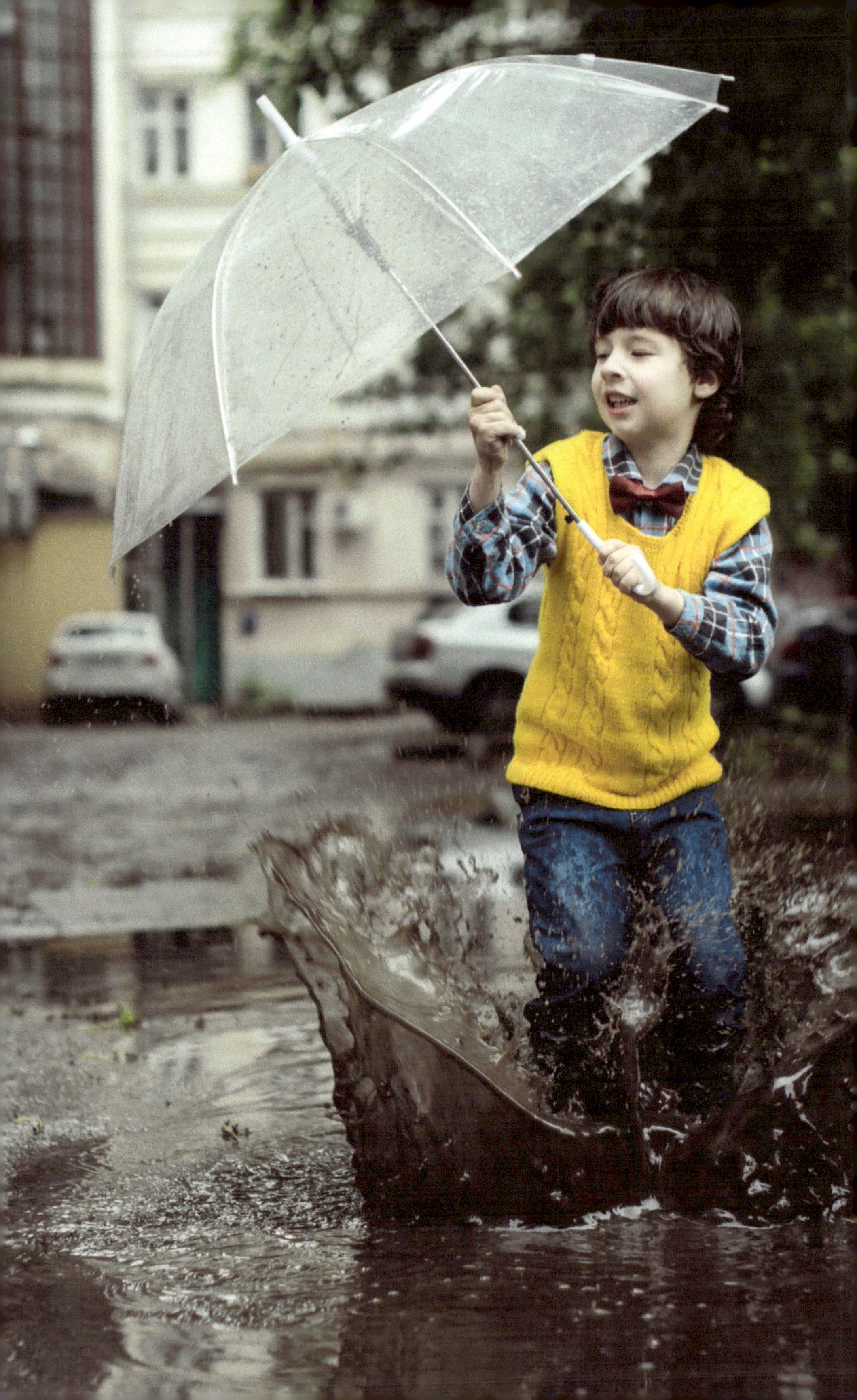

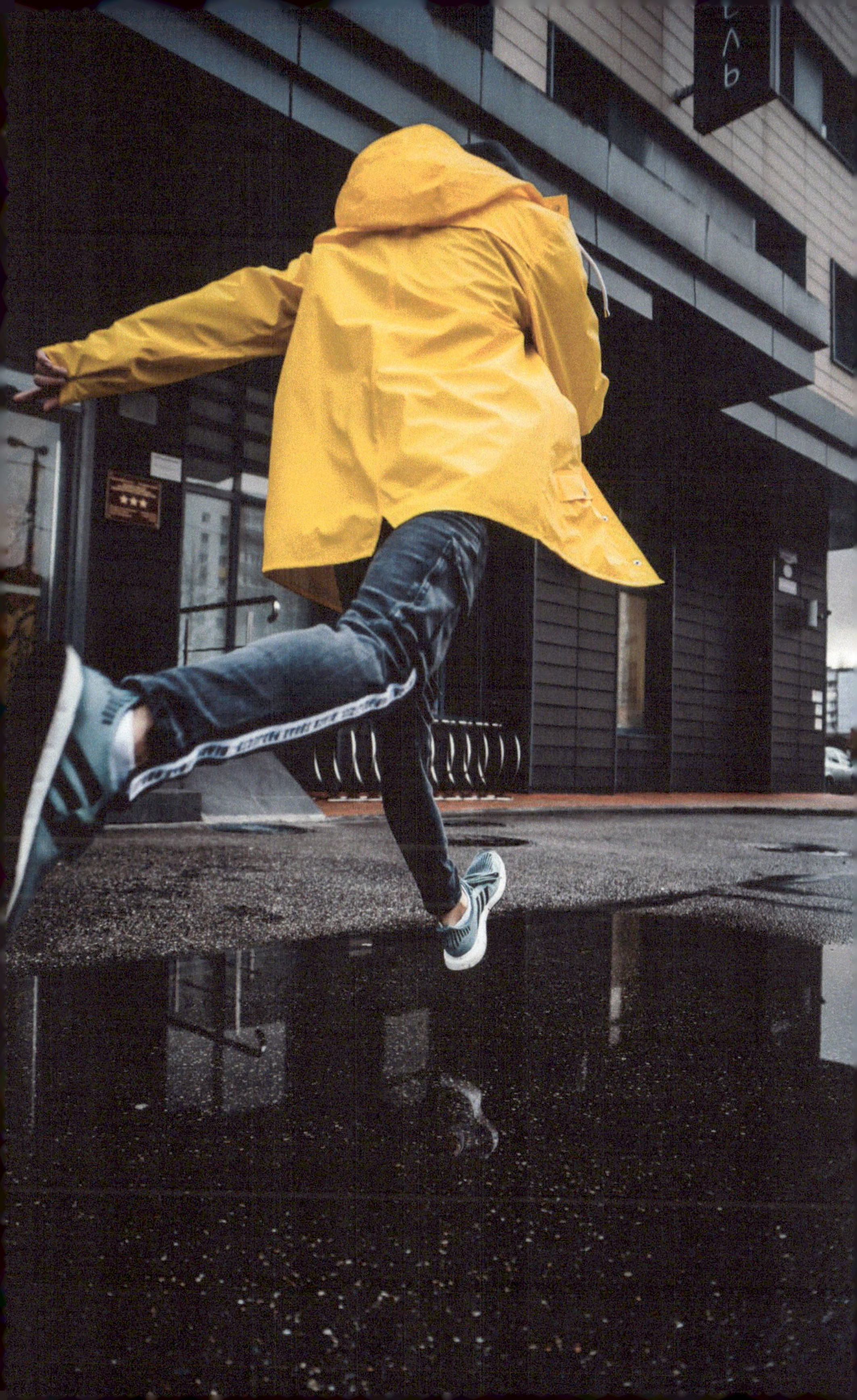

www.ingramcontent.com/pod-product-compliance
Lightning Source LLC
Chambersburg PA
CBHW040252220526
45473CB00001B/454
* 9 7 9 8 3 3 9 8 8 1 2 4 7 *